ACTION
SPEAKS
LOUDER

ABOUT THE AUTHORS

A. Jane Remocker is a graduate of the Dorset House School of Occupational Therapy, Oxford, England, and of the University of British Columbia, Canada. She has many years' experience in a variety of psychiatric settings and is presently working in private practice specializing in paediatrics. She has been responsible for setting up programmes in an acute-care hospital, a daycare programme and community workshop, and is widely experienced in working with groups of chronic psychiatric patients and the elderly in the community. She has served as a consultant to community-based organizations working with psychiatric patients, and to the Canadian Association of Occupational Therapists. Presently she works with school-age children who have delayed fine and gross motor skills, often with associated psychiatric problems.

Elizabeth T. Sherwood obtained her BA at the University of British Columbia and is a graduate of the Special School of Occupational Therapy, Kingston, Ontario, Canada. During her many years of clinical experience she has gained a reputation for being an expert in group techniques with psychiatric patients. She has worked with the physically handicapped and with psychiatric patients in acute-care hospitals (both in-patient and day care centres) in a chronic residential hospital, and in a community treatment centre. She has acted as a consultant in non-verbal techniques for both acute and chronic patients, and has been a guest lecturer at the School of Rehabilitation Medicine, University of British Columbia and at the School of Occupational Therapy at the Central Institute of Technology in Wellington, New Zealand. At present, she is a sole charge Occupational Therapist in a community-based mental health team and honorary Clinical Instructor at the University of British Columbia.

For Churchill Livingstone

Publisher: Mary Law
Project Manager: Valerie Burgess
Project Development Editor: Valerie Dearing
Design Direction: Judith Wright
Sales Promotion Executive: Hilary Brown

ACTION
SPEAKS
LOUDER

A Handbook of Structured Group Techniques

A. Jane Remocker BSR OT(C)
Occupational Therapist, Paediatric Private Practice and
Consultant to B C Children's Hospital, Vancouver, B C, Canada

Elizabeth T. Sherwood BA OT(C)
Sole Charge Occupational Therapist, Greater Vancouver
Mental Health Service, Vancouver, B C, Canada

Foreword by
Lila N. Quastel MA OT(C)
CEO and Consulting Occupational Therapist, Northwest
Rehabilitation Consulting and Management Services;
Assistant Professor Emerita, School of Rehabilitation Medicine,
Faculty of Medicine, University of British Columbia

SIXTH EDITION

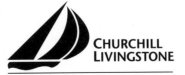

CHURCHILL LIVINGSTONE

EDINBURGH LONDON NEW YORK PHILADELPHIA SAN FRANCISCO
SYDNEY TORONTO AND TOKYO 1999

CHURCHILL LIVINGSTONE
An imprint of Harcourt Brace and Company Limited

First Edition 1977, published by A. Jane Remocker and Elizabeth T. Storch
Second Edition 1979
Third Edition 1982
Fourth Edition 1987
Fifth Edition 1992
Sixth Edition 1999

ISBN 0 443 058652

British Library Cataloguing in Publication Data
A catalogue record for this book is available from the British Library.

Library of Congress Cataloging in Publication Data
A catalog record for this book is available from the Library of Congress.

Note
Medical knowledge is constantly changing. As new information becomes available,
changes in treatment, procedures, equipment and the use of drugs become
necessary. The authors and the publishers have, as far as
it is possible, taken care to ensure that the information
given in this text is accurate and up-to-date. However,
readers are strongly advised to confirm that the information,
especially with regard to drug usage, complies with latest
legislation and standards of practice.

The
publisher's
policy is to use
**paper manufactured
from sustainable forests**

Produced by Addison Wesley Longman China Limited, Hong Kong
EPC/01

Foreword

Books should to one of these four ends conduce
For wisdom, piety, delight, or use.
John Denham

This little book is my old friend. I was a colleague of the authors at the time of its inception; I watched its growth and development, celebrated its publication and applauded its popularity. I have used it extensively with small groups of clients and introduced it to successive classes of occupational therapy students from 1977 to 1990. The old friend has endured the test of time because it meets not one, but three of the four ends proposed by John Denham: use, wisdom and delight.

The book is for people who help people to help themselves. It is for mental health workers who understand the healing effects of both doing and talking. It is not true that actions speak louder than words. Each has an equal potential to be harmful or helpful. Together, doing and communicating can be powerful therapeutic tools, if used with sensitivity. The techniques described in this book encourage the use of a delicate interplay of both actions and words in delightful group exercises. The layout is cookbook style for ease of access and use. Each group activity is described in detail, including materials, timing, procedures and problems for which the activity is recommended. Like a valued recipe, once the exercise becomes familiar, variations and innovations present themselves for repeated use. The chapter entitled *Some basic concepts* is packed with information for students and provides good reference for educators and clinicians.

The wisdom of this book lies in the attention to universal, enduring mental health concepts such as self-esteem, awareness of self and others and social interaction, etc. The experienced authors write with clarity, simplicity and insight about those states of being when people become locked into themselves, self-deprecating and uncommunicative. To assist another person out of such a state is an art, a science, an acquired skill. My old friend endures because the authors had the wisdom to provide practical guidance in the development of such skills.

This book is fun to read and use. Many of the exercises help people laugh at themselves and with each other. Try a debate about jelly beans or second-hand shoes; play the game of charades; or find out just who stole those cookies from the cookie jar. For wisdom, delight and use, this is a wonderful handbook of structured group techniques.

Minor changes occurred in the first four editions between 1977 and 1987. For the fifth edition, the authors expanded on the introductory content to include theoretical models of occupational therapy familiar to faculty, students and practitioners in the 1990s. In this new sixth edition there have been major changes in the exercises. Activities which originated in the 1970s, and were in popular use in that era, have been replaced by new exercises, many suitable for children. Occupational therapists working with children have, over the years, recognized the value of this book for pediatric populations and will applaud the changes in this sixth edition. In addition, considerably more emphasis has been placed on the nonverbal aspects of communication, in accord with recent research emphasizing the role played by body language in conveying meaning and in 'labelling' others as different.

In my foreword to the 1992 edition, I expressed the hope that this book would be around in the 21st century. How appropriate that the new edition coincides with the rapid approach of the year 2000. According to the authors this is their final edition. If that proves to be the case, the reader is advised to make sure they obtain copy. However, the book has proved to be widely used and the authors may well succumb to popular demand. I still expect this old friend of mine to be around and useful for many decades. Try it: you too will find yourself delighted.

Bookes give not wisdome where none was before,
But where some is, there reading makes it more.
Sir John Harrington

Vancouver, Canada, 1998   Lila Quastel

Preface

When we first wrote this book in 1977 we were both newly married, energetic young professionals, with 21 years' experience collectively in occupational therapy. The idea for the book evolved out of our clinical work in an acute-care teaching hospital, where some of our time was spent instructing other professionals and students on the effective use of structured group techniques. The book in its final form resulted from the merging of our two different cultural and educational perspectives – Betty's from Canada and Jane's from England.

Our families grew; our clinical experience widened and significant developments occurred in the fields of psychiatry and occupational therapy. In psychiatry there have been increasing developments in biochemical intervention. Patient populations have also changed due to a philosophy based on treating more people within their own community rather than in the hospital setting. Thus the patient population in acute-care hospitals tends to be more severely ill, whereas out-patient units and other community facilities are treating an ever-increasing number of chronic patients. With the growing importance of adequate social skills for the chronic patients and the rebuilding of self-esteem for the acutely-ill patients, structured groupwork is a valuable treatment mode to meet these needs.

The profession of occupational therapy has developed a clearer definition of its role in assessment and treatment in psychiatry. Assessment now is focused not merely on problems and strengths but also on the underlying causes. We have described two current paradigms of occupational therapy which represent different methods of assessing and treating a patient's functional state, using a specific frame of reference.

The sixth edition has given us an opportunity to listen to our readers and to make some of the changes they suggested as well as updating both the language and exercises to fit with current developments in psychiatric medicine. We have included exercises for children, regrouped the exercises for easier reference and emphasized the importance of nonverbal language skills as a critical part of communication.

We hope that these changes will be useful to therapists of all disciplines and take this book into the 21st century.

Vancouver, Canada 1998   E.T.S.
                                                                      A.J.R.

Acknowledgements

We developed *Action Speaks Louder* from our experience of working directly with patients, mostly in an acute-care psychiatric hospital, and without their participation and enthusiasm this book could not have been written. We were assisted and encouraged over the years by fellow professionals. Special thanks are due to Shirley Salomon BSR (OT), Desiree Betz BSR (OT), Lila Quastel MA OT(C), Tim Readman DipCOT PGEdDev OT(C), Aileen Stalker BSR (OT) MEd and M. Janette McMillan BSc MD FRCP(C).

This sixth edition, which will be published 20 years after the first one, was presented to us on disk. This not only presented us with an electronic challenge but also allowed us to make many changes much more easily. It offered us a chance to update the language and suggestion lists offered, as well as to remove a number of outdated exercises and introduce some new ones. Our readers asked us to group the exercises for easier reference, which we have done, including a new section that emphasizes nonverbal skills. We have also indicated the optimum number of participants for each exercise and whether it is suitable for use with children.

Lastly, we are grateful to our families, Geoff, Ben, Sara, Gail and Chris, for their cheerful patience with us during the book's conception and successive rebirths.

Contents

Introduction

In this manual you will find a collection of exercises which have been designed to help individuals feel more comfortable with themselves and others in a non-threatening group atmosphere. The self-awareness and skills which they gain will give them the strength to go out and not only meet other people but also experience more effective and satisfying communication.

The exercises have come to us as folk-songs come to the balladeer. Some of them have been handed down from person to person and, as a result, have become changed. Some exercises have been invented in order to solve a particular problem at hand and some have developed spontaneously from a previous exercise or from one aspect of a group's discussion.

We have compiled this book of techniques as a result of our own experiences working with small groups in a variety of psychiatric settings. Individuals in these groups, aside from their presenting symptoms, often seemed to exhibit one or more of the following:

– difficulty communicating effectively with others
– difficulty recognizing and expressing their feelings
– difficulty perceiving others and/or self accurately
– difficulty generating solutions to personal problems
– difficulty controlling the arousal of debilitating anxiety.

These people, often psychotic or extremely disturbed, were unable to function in group psychotherapy. It was necessary, therefore, to develop a different form of group therapy, one which addressed real and special needs through structured activity. This type of groupwork, where activities are designed specifically to address the functional level of the clients, creates a therapeutic environment which identifies and builds on the skills of each person, rather than on those which are lacking. In general, severely disturbed clients seem to respond better in these types of groups than in unstructured psychotherapy groups.[1,2] We have come to realize that the use of structured exercises has a far wider application than we originally envisaged. This is because the exercises provide an opportunity for learning new and more appropriate ways of relating, for learning about oneself and one's reactions to situations and for learning about other people. The key to their effectiveness, however, is that they are simple and enjoyable for the participants. The exercises are written in a form that can be adapted to suit the age, level of functioning and purpose of any group of people who meet together in order to improve their self-awareness and ability to interact.

The book contains over 50 exercises, suitable for use in structured groupwork. By using these exercises we hope the reader will acquire the philosophy, experience and confidence which are necessary to create new exercises more suited to the specific needs of the reader's own clientele.

LAYOUT   The manual has been designed as a practical textbook for the student interested in expanding his knowledge of structured group techniques and as a handy reference book for the graduate therapist or teacher. It has been organized to be read and used as one would a cookery book, and the essential ingredients, which should be considered before carrying out the procedure, are listed under the following headings:

Title. This is the descriptive heading which is designed to help the leader quickly recall the technique involved. For example, *Self-portrait collage* is an exercise in self-awareness.

Time. An approximate time allowance is given. This should be of assistance in the planning of a session, since it is important to know whether to use one exercise or several during the time available.

Group size. The number of participants given indicates the maximum recommended for the particular exercise. When it is also an appropriate exercise to use with a group of children, this is indicated. Six is the maximum number of children recommended, especially if several of them exhibit poor impulse control or hyperactivity.

Recommended for these problems. If the exercises in this book are to be constructive and appropriate they should be related specifically to the problems of the individuals in the group. The first thing to do, therefore, is to identify the problem areas and then choose exercises which relate to them. In each exercise the problems addressed have been identified and articulated in the language of two models of Occupational Therapy: Human Occupation[3] and Life-style Performance.[4] For easy reference the problems are listed separately for each model and alongside the appropriate sub-system, for example:

Human Occupation	*Life-style Performance*
Perf. Decreased concentration	Cog. Short attention span

The sub-systems of the Model of Human Occupation have been abbreviated as follows: Vol. (Volition), Hab. (Habituation), Perf. (Performance). The sub-systems of the Model of Life-style Performance have been abbreviated as follows: Sens/mo. (Sensory/motor), Cog. (Cognitive), Psyc. (Psychological), Intp. (Interpersonal). Several different problem areas can be focused upon in any one exercise.

Stage of group development. Under this heading we have indicated the degree of closeness in relationships which we feel should exist amongst the group members in order for the exercise to be appropriate. Whether an exercise is suitable or not for a particular group of people depends on many complex factors. The general statements we have made regarding suitability, therefore, should be used as a guideline only. In deciding whether to use an exercise or not, we feel the amount of interpersonal contact that is required by the exercise and the amount of interpersonal sharing that the group can actually tolerate are two very important factors.

Synopsis. Under this heading you will find a thumbnail sketch of the exercise. The synopsis is designed with two purposes in mind: first, that you, as the leader, can assess quickly whether the exercise is appropriate and, second, that once you are familiar with its title, you can recall the procedure easily.

Materials and equipment. In this section we have listed those things that need to be organized or prepared before starting an exercise. The materials required for some exercises include the preparation of a list of topics. Where this is necessary we have compiled some suggestions and these are found directly after the exercise The ideal setting has been indicated but this is a guide only.

Procedure. This section is divided in half longitudinally. On the left-hand side of the page is a step-by-step description of how the exercise can be presented. On the right-hand side of the page is an explanation of the therapeutic aspects of some of the steps, often in relation to the problems listed above.

Discussion topics. The discussion which follows participation in an exercise is an important part of the whole experience. In fact, the main purpose of some exercises is to stimulate conversation, which then allows a person to talk about his subjective reactions, hear the comments of others and consider how this experience relates to his daily life. For example, in the exercise *Masks,* if through the discussion an individual becomes interested in the difference between how he appears to others and how he feels, this information may be integrated into the belief system, resulting in new patterns of behaviour. In the Human Occupation Model this information is input, the integration is throughput, while the change in behaviour is output. In the Life-style Performance Model this awareness in the Psychological sub-system will cause changes in the area of the Interpersonal sub-system. Without a discussion, most of the exercises may appear purposeless to the participants and lack relevance to their problems. Under this heading in each exercise you will find a few ideas to present to your group members for their consideration.

Your variations. We have presented the exercises in their most basic and, therefore, structured format. For this reason they will not be suitable for all situations or all groups of people. The *Your variations* space is an opportunity to record personal observations regarding the effectiveness of a particular exercise, variations that could be tried and recommendations for the future.

The exercises in this book are grouped into four main types: self-discovery, verbal, nonverbal and becoming acquainted. They include a range of choices such as warm-ups and theatre games, as well as the use of music, art and familiar games.

Verbal exercises are techniques generally of a more intellectual and sedentary nature. They tend to focus on such complex verbal skills as being able to organize and express one's thoughts and opinions in a clear and concise manner (e.g. *Save yourself*), to recall past knowledge and obtain and use current information (e.g. *Newspaper quiz*), or to listen to others and ask questions (e.g. *Monologue or dialogue*). The exercises make use of words, both written and spoken, and provide enjoyable opportunities to practise conversation. The nonverbal paralinguistic skills of voice intonation, clarity, pitch and volume can also be addressed through these exercises. Generally the stimulation required to hold an individual's attention must come from within himself.

Nonverbal exercises on the other hand, are techniques which tend to promote body awareness, physical coordination, self-expression and social interaction. Generally the stimulation required to hold the individual's attention is external, provided by the group as a whole or by individuals or objects within it. Many of the exercises also provide an enjoyable opportunity for a person to experience social interaction of a kind which he might normally avoid. They enable people to loosen up with more basic instinctual and physical forms of self-expression such as body rhythm and movement and allow them to experience aspects of themselves which they may wish to explore, develop or change. The exercises can be used to help participants to develop both their receptive and their expressive nonverbal language skills. Exercises for developing a greater comfort level with the use of appropriate eye-contact, facial expression and gestures, touch, use of interpersonal space and rhythm are included.

Self-discovery exercises may be verbal or nonverbal in form. Through them people become aware of their feelings, beliefs, support network or the stressors in their lives. Some use projective techniques in which a product – drawing, collage, diagram – is made, often using symbols to express unconscious material. Since a person often feels inhibited when speaking, use has been made of various expressive media such as music, art and drama. These forms of creative expression enable a person to say something about himself at a time when he is still unable to express himself in words. The information gained through symbolic representation is long-lasting and leads to reclaiming internal locus of control and personal responsibility.

Becoming acquainted exercises may be of short duration, such as warm-ups, or they may last the entire session. They help people who do not know one another to become better acquainted. They often take the form of light-hearted games through which participants begin to feel comfortable with one another. They encourage the learning of names and what information is appropriate to share when getting to know people, as well as some subtle nonverbal skills such as becoming aware of and matching other people's rhythms. These exercises can be used to teach the basic skills required in getting to know people, as well as providing an atmosphere in which individuals can begin to look at other social communication problems in greater detail. Participants generally experience a positive interaction with one person or with the entire group.

Theatre games are simple, structured exercises of the kind often used by actors to improve their ability to think quickly, to be spontaneous, to improvise, to speak clearly, to trust others, to work in cooperation with others, to concentrate and to be decisive. The emphasis in most of them is upon clear, direct communication, whether it be verbal or nonverbal, and if they are used well they offer an excellent opportunity to practise, improve or change social behaviour in an enjoyable and accepting atmosphere.

Warm-up exercises are usually of short duration. They are used at the opening of a group to help the participants feel more comfortable with each other and to assist in the process of group cohesion.

In reading through the book and in carrying out the exercises described, it should be pointed out that exercises such as these will rarely be used in isolation. They are far more likely to be utilized as part of a person's total treatment programme, which may include such other things as chemotherapy, individual supportive psychotherapy, occupational therapy and recreational activities.

Finally, the book has been written to be used as a practical manual. We anticipate it will give ideas, stimulate the imagination and provide a creative method of approaching problems. However, it is only a beginning and we realize that there are areas which are, of necessity, brief. The Bibliography at the end of the book contains some excellent additional reading, together with books and journal articles offering many more ideas for structured groupwork. These books can be obtained from public libraries and, together with this handbook, will provide a firm basis for the reader to develop a larger and more personalized repertoire of exercises.

REFERENCES

1. Smith, P. B. (Ed.) (1980) *Small Groups and Personal Change*, p. 111. London: Methuen.
2. Kaplan, Kathy L. (1988) *Directive Group Therapy*. New Jersey: Slack.
3. Kielhofner, G. (Ed.) (1985) *A Model of Human Occupation, Theory and Application*. Baltimore: Williams & Wilkins.
4. Fidler, G. S. (1988) The Life-style Performance Profile. In: Robertson, Susan G. (Ed.) Focus: *Skills for Assessment and Treatment*. Section: Frames of Reference – Practice Models. Rockville, MD. American Occupational Therapy Association.

Some basic concepts

Over the past 10 years there have been remarkable pharmacologic advances in the treatment of psychotic disorders. At the same time there has been a trend in Canada to downsize the larger psychiatric institutions and treat the severely mentally ill person in the community. Deinstitutionalization results in the movement of individuals from an isolated environment to the broader social community and this means that the encouragement of socially appropriate behaviours through structured activities becomes vitally important.

In the past traditional neuroleptic medications were used to treat only the 'positive' symptoms of schizophrenia which include delusions, hallucinations, excitability, grandiosity and hostility. Now the atypical neuroleptics such as clozapine, risperidone and olanzapine relieve the physical burden of the side-effects of traditional neuroleptics, such as stiffness, dystonias, Parkinsonism and tardive dyskinesia. The new neuroleptics also help treat the 'negative' symptoms of schizophrenia which include social withdrawal, lack of motivation and spontaneity, poverty of speech, blunted affect, and lack of pleasure and ability to feel intimacy. The new specific serotonin reuptake inhibiting medicines make taking an antidepressant less onerous.

Using an approach which combines these medications and psychological, social and physical activity interventions we can look forward to significant improvements in the functioning of these individuals overall.

Much of this book is about being able to communicate, both about ourselves and with others. For many of our clients the onset of their mental illness interrupted the learning process in this area, which begins in early childhood and continues through adolescence into adulthood. Participation in exercises such as these offers the chance to learn or relearn basic communication skills in a safe and supportive setting.

Communication requires being able to speak, listen and interact with other people in order to share such things as attitudes, ideas, emotions and activities. It is a very complex and dynamic process requiring the use of both expressive and receptive skills and it is not nearly so simple as just being able to talk. When we speak (verbal communication) we also communicate continuously nonverbally through posture, facial expression, gestures, tone of voice, eye-contact and so-on. For most people these nonverbal acts are an entirely unconscious process but they are perceived by others as a very reliable indicator of how we actually feel. It follows, therefore, that if one is to communicate satisfactorily it is important to have both effective and appropriate verbal and nonverbal skills and to be able to synchronize the two.

If one has to place emphasis on one or other set of skills, research indicates that when words and nonverbal expression do not match it is the nonverbal information that is paid more attention to in most circumstances, rather than the words. When people make mistakes in speech, society tends to make judgements about their intellectual abilities and consider them perhaps uneducated or not so smart. In other words, we excuse them. If a person makes mistakes in nonverbal communication, society is far more likely to make a judgement about their mental stability and label them as weird, scary or unstable and, rather than excusing them, exclude them. The person may not even be aware that they are making nonverbal mistakes, but they will be aware of the results – social isolation, rejection and loneliness. Even such seemingly small nonverbal behaviours as habitually clearing one's throat, standing too close or speaking too loudly or in a monotonous voice can be cause for ongoing social rejection. This new edition of *Action Speaks Louder* includes more exercises that emphasize the use and/or development of receptive and expressive nonverbal communication skills.

Norwicki and Duke (1992)[1] identified six specific nonverbal language skills that they consider are at the root of many communication difficulties between individuals. These are rhythm and use of time, interpersonal distance and touch, gestures and posture, facial expressions, paralinguistics (voice, tone, pitch, etc.) and objectics (style of dress).

A person's internal rhythm is determined by many factors such as where they grew up, their cultural background and genetic predisposition. We all know people who label themselves as either morning or evening people, who are the same nationality as ourselves, who do things quickly or slowly or who speak in a particular manner. Whether we realize it or not there is a natural tendency for individuals to form relationships with those whose internal rhythm is similar to their own as being 'out of sync' can make a person feel anxious. It is a useful nonverbal skill, therefore, to become aware of one's own rhythm and that of others so that temporary adaptation can be made. Studies show that the most popular children and adolescents are those who can identify the internal rhythms of others and adapt their own to match for the duration of their interaction. Exercises involving the use of rhythm (e.g. *Movement and sound circle*) or matching movements with others (e.g. *Mirrors*) can be used to introduce this nonverbal skill.

The ability to use time appropriately is another useful nonverbal skill. Being able to organize one's day and carry out plans, either alone or with others, is the sign of an individual who has a well developed sense of internal locus of control. It also builds self-esteem by enabling the person to engage in fulfilling daily activities such as work and recreation and to build satisfying relationships. For the person who cannot use time appropriately the opposite is also true. Being habitually late for events, for example, can be interpreted by others as not caring enough and result in dismissal from employment or the ending of potentially rewarding friendships. An exercise such as *Time management* is excellent for helping individuals look at how they spend their time.

Interpersonal distance and understanding what it means in social situations is another nonverbal skill that affects our interpersonal relationships. Each person is surrounded by an invisible bubble of space, known as personal space, which other people can violate by coming too close. The size of this bubble varies from individual to individual and between cultures, and depends upon the social situation the individual finds herself in. All cultures have unwritten rules regarding interpersonal distance that people unconsciously adhere to and which vary according to the type of interaction which is occurring. When the rules are broken it may create social alienation for the individual and discomfort for all those involved. It is, therefore, important to understand and follow the rules that are present within one's own culture if one is to be socially accepted. The exercise *Am I too close or too far away?* is an excellent one for working on this skill.

How and where does one touch other people, so as to convey meaning accurately and not offend? Again there are clear but unwritten rules regarding this which vary depending on the nature of the interaction, the relationship of the individuals involved and the culture. In North America, for example, it is not appropriate to touch people in social situations on the front of the body. Touching on the shoulder is the most acceptable way to catch someone's attention, but since to do this one must violate the other person's personal bubble, it should be accompanied by saying 'excuse me'. Shaking hands is a socially acceptable form of greeting. When should one hug or kiss a person when greeting them? These and other rules regarding socially appropriate touching can be discussed following involvement in exercises such as *Caboose* and *Guided exploring*.

Using one's hands to make appropriate gestures requires both good expressive and receptive skills. Gestures are more elaborate in some cultures than others and are used to convey a multitude of meanings. Fingers, for example, can be used to emphasize speech, to welcome or to insult depending on which one is used and in what way. *Hand puppets* is an excellent exercise to explore the use and diversity of hand gestures and to practise synchronizing them with speech.

We use our body all the time to convey feelings which then influence those around us. A person's posture while sitting, standing, walking, etc. represents continuous unspoken dialogue and can be 'read' from close up or far away. Take, for example, the teacher who sits on the front of her desk to convey to her class that this will be a relaxed, informal session or who later stands behind her desk, leaning forward on her arms to convey the message 'listen carefully to what I am about to say'. We also need to become aware of the type of resting posture we assume when we are feeling neutral, since this may inaccurately communicate how we are feeling and result in negative consequences. In the exercise *Charades*, for example, different types of postures can be practised to convey different feelings and the importance of posture as a nonverbal skill can be discussed.

Research indicates that effective eye-contact and use of smiling are the two most frequently noted characteristics of socially successful children. We actually spend anywhere from 30% to 60% of the time looking at the faces of the people with whom we are interacting and if we do not look at them we miss valuable interpersonal information. Lack of eye-contact is often observed among people with mental illness and when they begin to initiate eye-contact it can be an indicator of the early stages of recovery. If a person has difficulty making and maintaining appropriate eye-contact it can cause others to think the person is not interested in them or in what is going on. This can cause problems socially. It is also important to look at a person in order to read their facial expression, gestures, posture, etc. so that one can react appropriately. Reading faces though is only half of the story; we also have to produce facial expressions that reveal our true feelings. Exercises such as *Masks* or *Mirrors* offer opportunities to practise and discuss these skills.

Paralanguage, or all the sounds that either accompany spoken language or act instead of words to communicate emotion, is another important aspect of nonverbal communication. The sound patterns we use, the speed at which we talk, the tone, volume and pitch of our voices and the ability to synchronize these with words all affect the quality and quantity of our social interactions. Constantly clearing one's throat or a high-pitched laugh are examples of expressive para-linguistic problems which can lead to social rejection. Rapid speech can have an irritating or intimidating effect, slow speech can be soothing or be seen to signify insecurity. Exercises such as *Soapbox, Story-telling* or *Monologue or dialogue* are enjoyable ways to practise and improve paralinguistic skills.

The way we dress, the type of jewellery we wear, our hairstyle and so on is an important form of nonverbal communication called objectics. Looking after one's personal hygiene and wearing clean, laundered clothing can be important or rather lack of attention to these things may have disastrous social consequences for the person involved and is often due to lack of awareness. However, these issues are dealt with best on a one-to-one basis and are not addressed in this book.

When preparing and leading any kind of structured group therapy there are many aspects that should be taken into consideration. We would like to share some of the concepts that we have learned as a result of our experience working with groups.

PLANNING   It is very important to allow sufficient time for preparation. The group leader needs to prepare not only the equipment and materials required but also to give thought to the focus, choice of exercises, etc. In order to do this effectively the following points should be considered:

Location and time When planning a programme of structured group techniques consider where the session should be held and at what time. Consistent time and location are very important and enable the participant to incorporate the group into his daily routine with ease. Even if one plans to use a different location for a particular session it is far better to meet at the usual location and move on from there. This is particularly true when the participants are travelling from their homes in order to attend.

A few exercises lend themselves to being done out of doors and, in fact, being taken out of their usual setting may stimulate the participants to perceive a familiar experience from a completely different perspective. Three factors which make it inadvisable to hold a group outside are: (1) if the exercise requires considerable concentration, (2) if the group contains some people who are easily distracted, and (3) if the group contains members who are on medication which makes them sensitive to the ultraviolet rays of the sun.

Usually the exercise and the discussion period following an exercise will be carried out in one location. There are times, however, when this is not advisable, for example, when the energy level of the group is very low. If this occurs, a break can be introduced by moving to another room and carrying out the discussion over coffee and cookies. Talking while eating is not only easier, but also tends to unite a group of people and to help them feel more comfortable with one another.

Whatever facilities are available, it is important to remember that the suitability of the chosen environment will impact directly on the effectiveness of the exercises.

Use of space The features of the space where the group is going to be held should be considered when choosing the location, since this factor can encourage or discourage relaxed interaction between people. The space can be considered from three separate perspectives: the fixed-feature space, the semi-fixed feature space and the informal space.[2]

Fixed-feature space refers to the immovable boundaries, such as the walls, windows and doors. Since these features cannot be changed it is important to choose a room that is large or small enough to do the group exercises in comfortably.

Semi-fixed feature space is that which is organized by the movable objects within the room, such as the tables and chairs. People tend, either consciously or unconsciously, to assign meaning to both the fixed and semi-fixed features and respond accordingly.

When arranging the table(s) and chairs for a structured group activity it is important to consider the type of interaction you wish to encourage and how you wish the group members to be oriented, one to another. When the semi-fixed features of space are arranged so as to encourage interaction this is called 'sociopetal'. When they are arranged to discourage interaction it is known as 'sociofugal'.[3] The most sociopetal position for two people is when they are face to face; a much less sociopetal position is when they stand side by side at 180° to one another. For most group activities we prefer either the first position or somewhere between the two, such as is achieved by sitting group members in a circle, so they can see every other member without too much effort.

If the activity requires that a table or tables be used, the arrangement of the group members around the table can foster or inhibit interaction. Figure 1 shows a table arrangement for eight people. When such a seating plan is used the person at the 'head' of the table usually emerges as the leader. Consider whether you as the group leader wish to take this position or perhaps assign it to a group member whom you wish to encourage to take a leadership role. In a seating arrangement such as this there are also 'hot spot seats' where the participants tend to talk more. The two ends of the table and the two middle positions generate participation, so the amount of participation by each individual can be influenced to some degree by where he sits.[4]

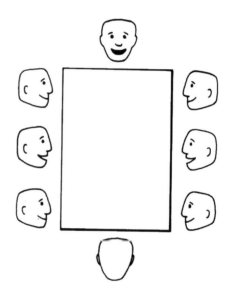

Fig. 1

If you observe people in different social situations you will notice that they tend to choose different seating arrangements for different types of interaction. For comfortable conversation people like to sit at the corner of a table (Fig. 2a). If two people are working together on a task the side-by-side position is one they prefer (Fig. 2b), whereas, in competitive tasks, the participants often choose to sit across from one another (Fig. 2c).

Many structured group exercises suggest a more informal seating arrangement. Placing the chairs in a circle (Fig. 3a) or horseshoe arrangement (Fig. 3b) is a suitable solution. In the first arrangement each position encourages an equal amount of participation and the leader's position is not emphasized. In the horseshoe the leader sits slightly

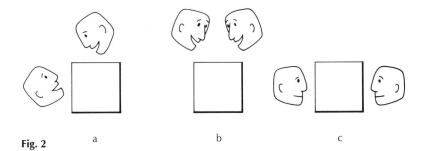

Fig. 2   a   b   c

apart and, thereby, emphasizes his position of control.[5] Organizing the seating arrangement is, therefore, a very important part of the preparation of structured groups.

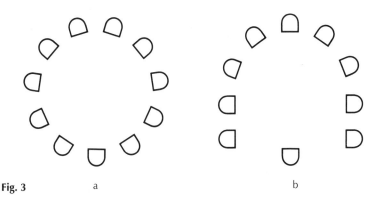

Fig. 3   a   b

The third kind of space to be considered is informal space. This is the space that surrounds each person. It can be thought of as a 'bubble' of air, the size of which varies for each one of us and for every different situation in which we find ourselves. It has been determined that each cultural group uses specific distances for specific types of interaction and that these vary between cultures.[6] When introducing exercises that require the participants to be physically close, be aware that for some the invasion of their personal space may cause considerable anxiety. An example is the exercise *Mirrors*. Some people can maintain eye-contact while standing very close, whereas others find it makes them feel uncomfortable but will manage the exercise if they can back away to a comfortable distance.

Size of the group Obviously this is an important factor because some exercises are more effective when used with a large group of people and others are more suited to a small group. For example, many of the Theatre games require an audience component. Other exercises, such as *Compliments*, would take too long if the group were large and everyone was to take a turn. We find the optimum size for a structured group is eight to ten people, including staff.

If the membership of a structured group is small, e.g. five people including staff, we have noticed in practice that the participants may become anxious and reluctant to attend, as the staff–patient ratio is too high. With this size of group, video-replay techniques can be used to advantage since there is time available to record and watch the tape and use it as a reference for discussion (see section on Video-replay techniques, p. 25). However, it is possible to adapt and structure an exercise so that it can be done with two or three people just as effectively as with ten.

On the other hand, if a group is very large then it can be extremely difficult to help the quiet, withdrawn person to become involved. It is sometimes best to split a large group into smaller units, or structure the session so that the quiet members have an opportunity to join in.

Level of group cohesion

It is quite difficult to ascertain accurately the level of group cohesion but this can be assessed by considering: 'How long has the group been meeting together?'; 'How well do the group members relate to one another?'; 'How comfortable are they in group situations?'; 'Do they trust one another?'; 'Do they take an interest in or support one another?'; and 'Can they risk expressing their feelings to one another?'

Consideration of the above questions assists in determining which exercises are suitable, since each one varies in the amount of interaction and personal sharing that it requires. For example, if a group is meeting together for the first time it is unlikely that the people in it will feel able to share intimate problems. It would be much more suitable to focus the session on becoming acquainted and to utilize some exercises which would help the participants do this easily. In general, structured exercises, and particularly those with a nonverbal component, enhance warmth, trust and cohesion within a group, as long as they are used appropriately and in a manner which is acceptable to the participants.[7]

Levels of concentration

Every person in a group will be able to concentrate for a different length of time. Assessing this variable will help determine both which exercises are appropriate and also how many to use. A person's concentration tends to improve if he is truly interested in what is happening and if he is constantly involved and stimulated. This can be achieved if he is actively doing something or if he is given a part in the proceedings. Therefore, in a group where the majority of people have difficulty concentrating, it is usually advisable to use several exercises and to choose ones which are active rather than sedentary.

Needs of each person

In any group, each person will have his own particular problems. These are the problems that you will have identified in your initial assessment. These become translated into the goals that the person hopes to achieve or work towards while participating in appropriate exercises. Whereas the Human Occupation Model refers to them as 'patient problems' or 'treatment criteria', the Life-style Performance Model refers to them as 'skill deficiencies'.

This is always the first thing to think about, because it makes it possible to choose a focus for the session. The focus will probably be problem-related but where possible should be expressed in positive terms. For example, if one of the problems is that most of the people in the group have a diminished sense of personal effectivenes or loss of self-reliance, then the focus of the session could be building self-confidence.

We find that a focus helps people work on specific problems while giving them a sense of doing something which is both purposeful and constructive.

Frames of reference In the past, occupational therapists have applied a wide range of psychological theories to their practice. As a result of rapid changes in the profession there has been a growing movement to define and articulate specific occupational therapy frames of reference that are distinct from psychological theories.[8]

Several frames of reference have emerged and this book refers to the following two: the Model of Human Occupation by Kielhofner and the Model of Life-style Performance by Fidler.[9, 10]

Model of Human Occupation The Model of Human Occupation draws upon concepts from systems theory. It views every individual as an 'open system' in constant inter-action with the environment. How the person functions is determined by the state of his internal organization, of his external environment, or, more usually, a combination of both. The internal organization of a person can be determined by assessing the three sub-systems of Volition, Habituation and Performance and their interrelationships. Assessment of these sub-systems must recognize that they are concep-tualized as existing in a hierarchical relationship to one another (for example, Volition is constrained where deficiencies exist in the other sub-systems, whereas problems with Volition disorganize Habituation and Performance levels). The Volition sub-system is responsible for choosing and initiating occupational behaviour; the Habituation sub-system organizes occupational behaviour into patterns or routines; and the Performance sub-system is responsible for producing occupational behaviour.

Dysfunction of any one of the sub-systems can cause problems at another level. For example, ulcers are caused by an overstimulated parasympathetic nervous system (Performance sub-system) due to patterns of overwork (Habituation sub-system) and high stress and competition in the workplace (Volition sub-system).

A person, however conceptualized, does not exist in a vacuum. By viewing a person as an 'open system', the Model of Human Occupation recognizes that an individual is in constant interaction with the physical and social environment. Behaviour is maintained or changed through the cyclical process of intake, throughput, output and feedback. An individual's actions are considered to be the output of the human system. Feedback is provided by the consequences of these actions and this information is received by the person as intake. Throughput has already been discussed as the person's ability to process information based on the internal state of organization. For example, in the exercise *Soapbox*, each person in the group makes decisions about the chosen topic based on past knowledge and experience (intake); from this he then formulates and presents his ideas to the group (output); the response of the other group members, both verbally and nonverbally, will give information about his performance (feedback); feeling good about clearly stating his ideas to others gives a person confidence to express himself in social situations in the future (throughput).

Throughput can affect the three sub-systems in different ways. It affects Volition by reinforcing the individual's belief that expressing opinions is enjoyable, which will increase the likelihood that he will share his opinions with others more often. It affects Habituation because, having experienced success in formulating and verbalizing his ideas, the view that he held of himself of not being interesting to listen to or not being able to think clearly becomes invalid, resulting in more frequent exchanges of ideas with his friends. It affects Performance because, as the individual formulated and shared his opinions socially, the feedback of what works and what does not is incorporated into the self-image that guides his performance, and his skills improve.

Treatment and the selection of suitable exercises are also guided by the principles of systems theory and are based on rules of hierarchy:

1. *Higher levels guide lower levels.* This means that when planning a structured group one should focus on the highest level, in this case the Volitional sub-system, by taking into account a person's motivation, interest, goals, self-confidence and values when selecting activities.
2. *Lower levels constrain higher levels.* Structured group therapy should be organized at the lowest level, which would be the Performance sub-system. By developing basic skills at this particular level, change can be effected at the higher levels of Habituation or Volition.
3. *Dysfunction affects all levels.* Structured groupwork should focus on all three levels by using the high levels to assist and compensate for lack of skills at the lower levels. For example, an individual who has lost some short-term memory (Performance) can, through an exercise like *Name recall*, learn techniques for remembering names through association (Habituation).

The Model of Human Occupation is an excellent one to use in conjunction with the exercises offered in this book since it emphasizes the concepts of adaptive behaviour, change through action, the importance of social and/or environmental interaction and motivation.[11]

Model of Life-style Performance   In this model Fidler defines a person's performance as 'the ability to master roles and tasks of living that are essential to achieving social efficacy and personal satisfaction'.[12] The overall purpose of intervention, therefore, is to improve a person's performance in the areas of work, play and self-maintenance.

The model identifies four separate skill clusters:

1. self-care activity
2. personal needs satisfaction
3. contributions to the welfare of others
4. reciprocal interpersonal relationships.

It also presents a structure for organizing and identifying performance skills and deficits. Fidler suggests the information be collected through an interview tool called the Life-style Performance Profile.

The Model of Life-style Performance proposes four component systems of performance, Sensory-motor, Cognitive, Psychological and Interpersonal. Each must be examined in order to formulate a treatment plan, and acquisition of skills in any one of the component systems will be influenced by a person's age, cultural heritage, environmental demands and personal experience.

Occupational Therapy, using this model, 'is conceptualized as the process of using psychomotor activity to elicit those adaptive responses that support and enable the learning of performance skill'. In *Action Speaks Louder* the exercises offer an opportunity to practise psychomotor activity in an enjoyable and constructive way. Exercises should be analysed and selected for their appropriateness, which means that each exercise's Sensory-motor, Cognitive, Psychological and Interpersonal components are matched with each person's problems, strengths, values and ability to learn and change.

Choice of exercises When choosing appropriate exercises for a structured group many issues need to be considered and careful evaluation of the communication difficulties, both verbal and nonverbal, of each of the group members must be undergone. This assessment should also identify whether the specific deficits are expressive, receptive or a combination. Other considerations when selecting exercises should include the type of exercise, the level of physical activity it requires and whether the exercise(s) should be theme-related from day to day or just within the session.

Using the Model of Human Occupation, activities are selected for the level of arousal, exploratory behaviour, acceptance or achievement that is required to encourage active participation on behalf of the patient. The role, therefore, of the occupational therapist is to analyse the organizational status of all systems and sub-systems and to plan exercises that are meaningful and productive.

Using the Life-style Performance Model, exercises should be selected to provide an opportunity for the patient to participate in activities which will remedy or compensate for deficits and teach performance skills. The exercises chosen should address the specific areas of dysfunction and recognize existing strengths and resources. The patient's readiness to respond will depend upon his age, cultural background, economic and environmental resources.

In order to assist you to plan an effective group session, the exercises and problems/skill deficits have been cross-referenced in the index and are grouped according to the sub-systems they address in the two Models (Appendices A and B). Warm-up exercises are indicated to assist with the selection and sequencing of exercises. For further clarification, the sub-systems have been defined in the Glossary.

Once these aspects of planning a group have been considered, it is possible to put together a treatment programme that suits the needs of the individuals who will be participating, reflects the general functioning level of the group and is flexible. The flexibility is vital since it will allow the opportunity for the programme to develop in a new or unexpected direction initiated by the participants rather than by the group leader.

There are some specific problems that participants may experience which contraindicate the choice of certain exercises. For example:

- incapacitating side-effects of medication on an individual, such as tremor, blurred vision, Parkinsonism and dry mouth (contraindicated would be an exercise such as *Simultaneous conversations*)
- individuals with low ego-strength but high I.Q., i.e. those who are demoralized by their diminished ability to think and who feel 'put down' by being asked to participate in exercises which they feel are simple and childish (contraindicated would be *Newspaper quiz*)
- the over-active person who is extremely easily stimulated and has a tendency to interrupt or be disruptive (contraindicated would be *Movement and sound circle* or *Soapbox*)
- the suspicious person whose suspiciousness may tend to be increased by the nature of the exercise (contraindicated would be *Compliments*).

Lastly, always choose exercises with which you yourself feel confident and comfortable, since your own involvement and enthusiasm will tend to inspire the group members. The experience should be an enjoyable and worthwhile one for everybody involved.

PRESENTATION   Once the needs of each individual have been assessed and the skill deficits identified, thought should be given to the overall manner in which the exercise or exercises are to be presented.

In an inpatient setting, structured group treatment is the most effective method of presentation.[13] In order to accommodate a fluctuating population of patients in various stages of acute illness, treatment groups tend to be more effective using a supportive psychotherapeutic approach which allows skills to be addressed in a single session. In an outpatient setting a psychoeducational approach can be used, as the patient's illness has stabilized to a large extent, and patients are in a position to commit their attendance to a series of sessions. This method of presentation allows for skills to be taught in a single lesson or in a course of several lessons and is a very acceptable approach for patients, referring professionals and the group leader.[14]

Opening the group   Open each session with the name of the group, e.g. 'Good morning, this is the Self-esteem Group', so as to orientate those members who are confused and not quite ready to concentrate on the exercise at hand. Then introduce yourself and your co-therapist and ask the members in turn to introduce themselves. Or, if there is only one new member joining the group, ask the members to introduce themselves to him. Following this, give a few statements to introduce the general theme and explain the purpose of the specific exercises. It ensures that the session gets off to a good start by alleviating the initial apprehension that most people attending are likely to experience and helps the group members consider why they are there and what they might hope to learn. The introduction reinforces the importance of participating actively in the exercises.

Structured groupwork provides an experiential and enjoyable process, which is the essence of learning and behavioural change. Participation in purposeful activity is an effective aspect of a patient's treatment plan.

Presenting the exercise   The method of presentation can, and should, be varied, depending on the purpose of the exercise and the needs of the people in the group. For example, a group of students in a training session would need a far less simplified explanation than a group of young children or very withdrawn patients.

The therapist should begin by stating clearly the procedure and purpose of the exercise. When giving instructions, it is important to be aware of making them as explicit and concise as possible. The therapist should always enquire before commencing the exercise if everyone has understood the instructions correctly and be prepared to re-state specific points if there was anyone who did not follow all of them. This will provide an opportunity for points to be clarified, and give the person who is unassertive a chance to say he does not understand a particular part of the procedure. Once it has been ascertained that everyone has understood the steps in the procedure, the therapist is then in a better position to assess everyone's participation objectively. The job of re-stating is best done by the co-therapist since he, as a listener, is probably more conscious of any ambiguity.

The leader must know the directions of an exercise well and present them in a positive, assured manner. Some exercises can appear silly or childish if the group's confidence is not gained. Present them in such a way that their usefulness becomes apparent (e.g. as a tool for greater self-awareness and for direct communication). The therapist should also communicate nonverbally with body movements to clarify instructions and invite people to take part in the exercise.

The leader can explain the purpose of an exercise when introducing it (e.g. 'We are going to do an exercise to help you feel more comfortable expressing yourself in front of others'). However, sometimes it is better to move quickly from one exercise to another without any explanation in order to maintain the energy momentum. As the leader you must know the purpose of each exercise, but allow the participants to experience each one spontaneously without any pre-judgement. A discussion can always be held afterwards.

Roles   One important issue which determines the success of a group session is the whole question of leadership and roles.

Initially, leadership is usually assumed by the therapist or teacher. If you are working with another staff member, that person becomes your co-therapist. Both the leader and the co-therapist need to be actively involved in structured groupwork. For example, they should:

– participate fully in all parts of an exercise, acting as role-models
– volunteer personal information, enabling the group members to get to know them better
– be ready to volunteer ideas if the group members are passive
– be aware of everyone in the group and prepared to assist them individually to participate
– be ready to move on to another exercise at any time if the group members become restless or lose interest
– avoid sitting next to each other
– lead the discussion following an exercise, having given consideration to the focus and how it can be related to the daily lives of the patients
– encourage group members to make choices and decisions
– be prepared to hand the leadership over to a group member or members whenever it is appropriate.

Sharing the leadership amongst group members can be achieved by choosing exercises which call for a series of leaders. For example, in *Movement and sound circle* the leader chooses another person to succeed him, in *Word circle* the leadership is taken over by the person who loses the game and in *Mirrors* leadership alternates between partners.

It is also very important to allow individuals as many opportunities as possible to make decisions within the group setting. The reason for this is that it has been shown that this can affect both self-perception and a sense of competency in a positive manner.[15]

During exercises which are primarily verbal, such as *Simultaneous conversations*, and during any of the discussion periods, the leader and co-therapist have these additional duties: to equalize, to focus and to link-up.

To equalize is to assist everyone to participate more or less equally. This means that the therapist must first become aware not only of those in the group who tend to monopolize the conversation but also of those who quietly withdraw from it. He must then attempt to bring the quiet people into the conversation, using the topic as a means of entry. The therapist can re-channel the comments of those who are tending to monopolize by repeating or re-stating what the talkative person has said. Then the therapist can relate it to the topic and direct a question to one of the quieter members, thus inviting him to take part.

To focus is to be aware of the topic at all times and to help the group members from being side-tracked.

To link-up the leader must listen carefully to what is being said and, where necessary, re-state what one person has said to another person, pointing out where their ideas or experiences are similar. The purpose is to help the participants learn to listen and talk to one another, rather than always directing their comments to you, the therapist. The leader must be careful not to monopolize the conversation. A recent study with chronic schizophrenics suggests that person to person interaction may be altered to some degree by the amount of prompting done by the group leader. The results of this study indicated that if the group leader delays prompting group members by about 10–15 seconds, this will in turn encourage the members to prompt one another.[16]

Leadership There is a good deal of evidence that leaders of groups are highly influential. How does a therapist become an effective leader and what are the components of behaviour that contribute to that effectiveness?[17]

Lieberman et al. (1973), in their research, concluded that four attributes of leader behaviour were identifiable. These were emotional stimulation, caring, meaning attribution and executive function. Emotional stimulation describes leader behaviour which emphasizes revealing feelings, confrontation and challenging by both the leader and the group members. Caring refers to the giving of genuine praise, affection and support in order to foster positive feedback between group members during the exercises. Throughout the session acknowledge the positive contributions of group members to help them feel valued. Meaning attribution involves interpreting behaviour and providing frameworks for change, whereas executive function is defined in terms of such behaviours as setting goals or directions of movement, managing time, questioning, interceding, setting limits and encouraging decision-making.[18]

Results of research as to which components of leadership behaviour are most important are not conclusive; however, all authors agree that an element of support and caring is essential. Within the framework of structured groupwork this aspect of being a leader is particularly necessary[19] whereas emotional stimulation, with its attendant confrontation, should be emphasized the least. The nature of structured activities inevitably involves the leader in a great deal of organizing (executive function), particularly before the group meets. The activities themselves, if carefully chosen, tend to provide the medium for meaning attribution.

Many of the skills most strongly required of a good group leader are those very skills which are learned through experiences in groups. Thus it is suggested that the novice group leader should participate as a member in a variety of groups, seminars and discussions in order to develop a personal understanding of the group experience.[20] Working as a co-leader with an experienced leader, observing groups led by others and being observed leading groups, together with the all-important follow-up discussions about what occurred are also excellent ways to develop an effective leadership style.[21]

Subdividing a group   In some exercises the therapist has the choice of asking people to work in teams, in pairs or on their own. Division of a group into smaller units must be done with sensitivity and care, and there are many ways of going about it.

Teams   A team is a group of people who may or may not have a leader but who have a common purpose. Teams tend to be competitive, and can effect the following responses:

- increased motivation to participate
- increased involvement
- cooperation between members
- a sense of unity within the team because of a common opponent
- enthusiasm and goal-directed activity
- a sense of belonging to a smaller defined group.

A team is usually smaller in size than the regular group, which means that there are fewer people to relate to at any one time. This can be advantageous for the person who has great difficulty becoming involved with others.

Traditionally teams are formed by asking two people to be leaders and to choose their team members from the group. We find this method has very little value when working with people whose self-esteem is low, as the more popular members are chosen first, leaving someone with the feeling of rejection by being chosen last. Perhaps the simplest and most efficient method is to number off the participants 'one, two, one, two' and then ask them to form a team with all the other number ones, or number twos respectively. One can also arbitrarily split a group according to seating arrangement into smaller units. The last way, if you do not wish to use any of the above methods of team formation, is to leave the initiative to the group. Suggest they form into two equal teams with an even number of men and women on each.

Pairs   A pair is two people who are associated together. The situation where one person must work closely with another person during part of an exercise has many positive aspects:

- joint decision-making
- direct interaction with a specific person
- mutual support and ideas
- cooperation
- the sharing of information, experiences and feelings
- caring or taking responsibility for someone specific.

For the person who is very uncomfortable relating to a group of people, providing an opportunity in which he can start by relating to just one person is an excellent beginning. Two people constitute the smallest group and this tiny unit can always be enlarged slowly by structuring the situation (e.g. each pair joins another pair to make a foursome, and so on, until the whole group is reformed).

To divide a group into pairs one can invite each person to pair up with the person next to them, or give specific instructions such as 'Choose the person whom you feel you know best to be your partner' (appropriate for *Guided exploring*, p. 147), or, 'Choose the person whom you know least to be your partner' (appropriate for *Introductions*, p. 37)

Individuals A person on his own can be very strong or very vulnerable. Many of the people we see in hospitals are often extremely isolated. They have withdrawn from society and exist without much contact with others. An exercise in which someone participates on his own for part of the time is aimed at helping him see his potential as an individual in relation to those around him. Choose exercises carefully so that each person can participate as best he can, without feeling a failure. Avoid pointing out a person's weaknesses in front of others, since he is probably well aware of them already. Instead, concentrate on assisting him to acknowledge his strengths. Working on one's own can offer the following opportunities:

– to see one's ideas put into effect
– to make decisions
– to take on responsibility
– to share and care for others
– to lead
– to look objectively at oneself, both strengths and weaknesses
– to improve skills
– to experience success
– to become more self-confident
– to realize the effect of one's actions upon others.

In summary then, whether you choose to have the group members work alone, in pairs or in teams, make this decision on the basis of their needs and abilities.

Discussion period The discussion following an exercise is an important time. It is an opportunity to discuss something that has just happened and to begin putting the feelings experienced into words. The problems that a patient encounters during an exercise are often similar to those he experiences during his daily life. The discussion can be used to look more objectively at these difficulties.

The role of the therapist during the discussion is to have some questions prepared to stimulate conversation and to assist the members in expressing their experiences and feelings during the exercise.

Most people have some difficulty sharing their personal experiences in a group setting. There are various ways in which a therapist can make this easier for everyone concerned. For example, the people participating may feel more relaxed about talking if they are sitting around a small table, or are seated in a small room on some comfortable cushions talking over a cup of coffee.

It is important for the therapist to act as a role-model by being prepared not only to participate in exercises but also to share some aspects of his own experiences. It is necessary only to relate information that you are comfortable sharing and, where possible, to express your precise feelings briefly rather than enter into a descriptive story of events and thoughts. No doubt some people will question the rationale behind this statement, maintaining that a therapist should remain uninvolved if he is to be effective. This is definitely true in some circumstances; however, in our experience this model is not true when utilizing exercises such as these. Remaining uninvolved not only reinforces the thought, 'He's the therapist, I'm only the patient,' or 'He's the teacher, I'm only the student,' but it also impedes easy communication. By joining in, the therapist adds credibility to the exercise, enables the people in the group to relate to one another on a more equal basis and encourages more direct and open communication.

From our experience we have found that it is important to respect a person's right to withhold information and not share his feelings or reactions. A person will share his ideas and feelings when he is ready to do so.

Closing the group

Most groups are quite lively, requiring a high degree of physical and emotional involvement. After the last exercise it is important to bring the group together once more, both physically and mentally. Ask the members to re-form into one group, then summarize the theme for that day and indicate the key points that emerged from the exercises. Then ask the group to reflect for a moment on the session; the experience they have had and its value to them. After a brief quiet period invite each person to share his thoughts. Close the group on a positive note by describing briefly the topic for the next meeting and reminding everyone of the date, time and location.

Projective material

Material that the group members have produced can be displayed but only after you have obtained their permission to do so. These drawings or diagrams express, diagrammatically, some very sensitive areas in those members' lives and any wishes to keep this material private must be treated with respect.

Displayed drawings can often be used as a shorthand reference for yourself and the group members if the same subject matter occurs in a subsequent group. The picture will help quick recall of the information the group members conveyed. Group productions can also be displayed. This material gives each person a sense of belonging as it shows a joint effort, composed of contributions, representing the personalities of the members involved.

Video-replay techniques

Watching television is a common pastime for many people, making video television a familiar and acceptable medium to introduce into structured groupwork.[22] Its potential use is vast, limited really only by the availability and type of equipment and the creativity of the group leader. Some of the exercises in this manual are suitable for videotaping and, where we consider this to be so, we have included a footnote to this effect.

Taping a session can be done to provide the group with a visual and auditory record of the time they spent together. The tape can also be used as a very effective method of personal evaluation since the replay provides each person with an opportunity to look objectively at his own behaviour and to identify ineffective coping behaviours or defence mechanisms.[23]

We have used audiovisual replay techniques very successfully with exercises such as the ones in this book. Our experience, however, is that patients are often very anxious when the idea of taping a session is first brought up. We have learned, therefore, to introduce video-replay initially with exercises that are light-hearted (e.g. Theatre games such as *Action mime, Hand puppets, The matchbox is ...? or Simultaneous conversations*). The action and replay of these exercises is usually entertaining and does not necessarily have to be analysed. If the video-replay techniques are used with care and sensitivity then they can be extremely rewarding and informative for all the participants.

Video can also be used successfully as an instructional tool. Many patients have inadequate skills for coping with emotional states and feelings.[24] Tapes can be used very effectively to present scenarios to which the individual can respond and for teaching more appropriate ways of responding.

Social functioning in the community can be taught using the medium of video. A variety of public employees, such as bus drivers, policemen, shopkeepers, social workers, etc. can be taped in their place of employment, engaged in a typical dialogue with someone. Group members can view the interaction and practise questions and appropriate responses suitable for using in the community. Basic social skills, such as ritual greetings, how to begin and end conversations, how to give and receive compliments, etc. can also be shown using video. Role-playing situations or structured exercises can be used to reinforce learning.[25]

The medium of videotape can also be used creatively. The making of a videotape can provide an opportunity for the mastery of many skills and for expressing ideas. This approach has been used very successfully with adolescents.[26]

It is important for the therapist using video-replay to be very familiar with the equipment and its operation. This is because it is impossible to lead a group session calmly and perceptively if one is flustered and without half the necessary bits and pieces. It is also very important when using video-replay to ascertain from the group members that they are willing to have their group session taped.

EVALUATION   Once a group session is over, it is advisable to get together with the co-therapist and other staff members. This post-group meeting is the most advantageous time both to assess the group and to plan for the following session. During it, each group member, the group as a whole, the exercises used and any drawings or written material resulting should be given consideration.

Assessment of individuals   Throughout the exercises in the book we have listed, opposite the steps in the procedure, the usefulness of these steps in observing certain aspects of a person's behaviour. From these observations assessments can be made and some conclusions drawn about each participant's progress.

When using the Life-style Performance Model, observations should be recorded under the four sub-system categories of:

Sensory/motor:	Level of physical activity
	Coordination
	Spatial orientation
Cognitive:	Attention
	Memory
	Orientation
	Formulation of ideas
Psychological:	Mood
	Thought content
	Participation
	Expression of feelings
	Self-care
Interpersonal:	Verbal skills
	Nonverbal skills
	Cooperation
	Leadership skills
	Communication skills
	Trust

When using the Model of Human Occupation, the Directive Group Baseline Assessment Form (Fig. 4) is a useful tool. It provides a guide for focusing observations and for indicating strengths and weaknesses in each person's occupational functioning.

Evaluation of the group process   The group as a whole can be evaluated. Consider first the predominant feeling in the group (e.g. anger). If many of the members were angry, did you recognize it in time to use exercises that allowed the members to express or accept their anger? Did you initiate a discussion to help them investigate the cause of this anger? If the cause was known but the solution not attainable, did you use gross physical movement to allow an acceptable display of this anger? If you should have a similar mood in a future group, what would you change in order to handle it better?

DIRECTIVE GROUP
Baseline Assessment Form

Referral problem(s): #
S– (What patient said, characteristic statement)

O– PLEASE INDICATE APPROPRIATE RATINGS AND DESCRIPTIONS OF PATIENT'S BEHAVIOR:

	No	Partially	Yes	Not Observed
Basic Components of Volitional Sub-system				
• Patient identifies personal interests	1	2	3	X
• Patient demonstrates goal-directed behavior	1	2	3	X
• Patient demonstrates evidence of pleasure in activities, spontaneity, and anticipation of success.	1	2	3	X

Comments: (e.g. interests, goals, and motivation)

	No	Partially	Yes	Not Observed
Basic Role Behaviors				
• Patient participates actively in each activity	1	2	3	X
• Patient initiates one task-related comment/or makes one comment at a time	1	2	3	X
• Patient helps lead an activity	1	2	3	X

Comments: (e.g. manner/content of interaction, affect and coping skills)

	No	Partially	Yes	Not Observed
Basic Self-Maintenance Habits				
• Patient is dressed in street clothes prior to beginning of session	1	2	3	X
• Patient attends group on time	1	2	3	X

Comments: (e.g. appearance, response to time expectations)

	No	Partially	Yes	Not Observed
Basic Cognitive Skills				
• Patient is able to stay in session for duration of group	1	2	3	X
• Patient is able to focus attention for at least 25 minutes	1	2	3	X
• Patient is able to follow instructions on simple tasks	1	2	3	X
• Patient is able to explain directions	1	2	3	X

Comments: (e.g. fine, gross, and perceptual motor skills, elaborate on cognitive skills)

A– Assess patient's adaptive and maladaptive responses, areas of basic competence, comparison of current performance with past history, environmental requirements necessary to elicit adequate occupational behavior at this level.

P– Participate in the activities and relationships of Directive group for at least one week to work on the following short-term goal(s):

_____

Signature and Discipline's Initials

Fig. 4   Directive Group Baseline Assessment Form[27].

Then consider the participation of the group members. Did they take part or was there a sense of reluctance? Did they interact with one another or maintain their isolation? Was the energy generated by the group high or low? Did the group members lead the discussion or did you, as the therapist, have to initiate all the questions and comments? As a result of the work done during the session do you have a clear focus for the next group?

Evaluation of the exercises   This is the time to refer back to the focus of the group session and think about whether the exercises chosen were appropriate. Ask yourself if the session met your expectations as well as the needs of the participants. If not, was it that you chose inappropriate exercises or perhaps the appropriate ones but in an awkward sequence? Did you spend enough time warming up? Were the exercises active enough to involve all members? Were they too active, thereby excluding some people? Were they too intellectual? Was the content too abstract for the majority of the group members? Had the group evolved to a stage that allowed the members to share the feeling material you were seeking?

Think also about whether you were sufficiently well prepared and whether the location you chose was a good one. Were the exercises selected suitable for the number of people in the group and, finally, did you present the exercises in the most understandable way? If you can answer these questions you will learn from both your mistakes and your successes.

Group record   For your own reference you may wish to record the progress of each group. To be brief and concise, we suggest recording:

1. the date
2. the number of people who attended
3. the number of staff
4. the major goal or focus of the group
5. the mood of the group
6. the exercises used to obtain that goal
7. a good to bad rating scale of the success of each exercise with explanatory comments.

REFERENCES

1. Norwicki, S., Duke, M. (1992) *Helping the Child who Doesn't Fit In*. Atlanta: Peachtree Publishers.
2. Hall, E. T. (1966) *The Hidden Dimension*, pp. 95–105. New York: Doubleday.
3. Barnhart, S. A. (1976) *Introduction to Interpersonal Communication*, p. 95. New York: Thomas Y. Crowell.
4. Harrison, R. P. (1974) *Beyond Words: an introduction to nonverbal communication*, p. 153. New Jersey: Prentice Hall.
5. Harrison, R. P. (1974) *Beyond Words: an introduction to nonverbal communication*, p. 154. New Jersey: Prentice Hall.
6. Barnhart, S. A. (1976) *Introduction to Interpersonal Communication*, p. 97. New York: Thomas Y. Crowell.
7. Smith, P. B. (1980) *Group Processes and Personal Changes*, p. 144. London: Harper & Row.
8. Denton, Peggy (1987) *Psychiatric Occupational Therapy, A Workbook of Practical Skills*. Boston: Little, Brown.
9. Kielhofner, G. (Ed.) (1985) *A Model of Human Occupation, Theory and Application*. Baltimore: Williams & Wilkins.
10. Fidler, G. S. (1988) The Life-style Performance Profile. In: Robertson, Susan G. (Ed.) Focus: *Skills for Assessment and Treatment*. Section: Frames of Reference – Practice Models. Rockville, MD.
11. Kaplan, Kathy L. (1988) *Directive Group Therapy, Innovative Mental Health*

Treatment. New Jersey: Slack.

12. Fidler, G. S. (1988) *The Life-style Performance Profile.* In: Robertson, Susan G. Focus: *Skills for Assessment and Treatment.* Section: Frames of Reference – Practice Models. Rockville, MD.

13. Kaplan, K. L. (1988) *Directive Group Therapy.* New Jersey: Slack.

14. Lillie, M. D., Armstrong, H. E. Jr (1982) *Contributions to the Development of Psychoeducational Approaches to Mental Health Service.* American Journal of Occupational Therapy 36: 438–442.

15. Henry, A. D., Nelson, D. L., Duncombe, L. W. (1981) *Choice-making in Group and Individual Activities.* American Journal of Occupational Therapy 38: 245–251.

16. Turvey, A. A., Main C. J., McCartney, A. (1985) *Social Activity Groups with Chronic Schizophrenics: the influence of the therapist's behaviour.* British Journal of Occupational Therapy 48: 302–304.

17. Smith, P. B. (Ed.) (1980) *Group Processes and Personal Change,* pp. 81–100. London: Harper & Row.

18. Lieberman, M. A., Yalom, I. D., Miles, M. B. (1973) *Encounter Groups: first facts.* New York: Basic Books.

19. Smith, P. B. (Ed.) (1980) *Small Groups and Personal Change,* p. 113. London: Methuen.

20. Smith, P. B. (1980) *Group Processes and Personal Change,* pp. 81–100. London: Harper & Row.

21. Smith, P. B. (1980) *Group Processes and Personal Change,* pp. 198–205. London: Harper & Row.

22. Goldstein, N., Collins, T. (1982) *Making Videotapes: an activity for hospitalised adolescents.* American Journal of Occupational Therapy 36: 530–533.

23. Holm, M. B. (1983) *Video as a Medium in Occupational Therapy.* American Journal of Occupational Therapy 37: 531–534.

24. Denton, P. L. (1982) *Teaching Interpersonal Skills with Videotape.* Occupational Therapy in Mental Health 2: 17

25. Holm, M. B. (1983) *Video as a Medium in Occupational Therapy.* American Journal of Occupational Therapy 37: 531–534.

26. Goldstein, N., Collins, T. (1982) *Making Videotapes: an activity for hospitalised adolescents.* American Journal of Occupational Therapy 36: 530–533.

27. From Kaplan, K. L. (1988) *Directive Group Therapy,* p. 50. Thorofare, New Jersey: Slack.

EXERCISES

Exchanging chairs
(warm-up)

Allow 10 minutes
Group size: 10 adults/6 children

This is a *warm-up* technique which encourages body contact and concentration.

Recommended for these problems

Model of Human Occupation

Vol.
- feelings of powerlessness over personal actions resulting in apathy
- decreased belief in self as indicated by difficulty in social interactions

Perf.
- decreased concentration (5 minutes or less)
- slowing of perceptual-motor skills

Life-style Performance Model

Sens/mo. – slowed sensory-motor output
Cog. – short attention span
Psyc. – apathy
Intp. – limited interpersonal skills

Stage of group development

Use this exercise at the beginning of any group in which the members have great difficulty communicating with one another and in which the general mood is one of lethargy.

Synopsis

Two players exchange seats when their 'names' are called, while the caller attempts to sit in one of their vacated chairs.

Materials and equipment

Chairs in a circle.
Have one less chair than the number of people in the group.

Procedure

Ask each person to choose a vegetable.[1,2]	To initiate active participation.
Explain that the game will begin with one person standing in the centre of the group. He will call out two vegetables and those two people must	People who have slow psychomotor skills and are left standing without a chair to sit on are rewarded by taking the leadership position of caller.

1. For people whose concentration is very poor allow each person to write the vegetable he has chosen on a piece of paper and then pin it to his chest.
   An alternative to this would be to list the vegetables chosen on a blackboard, as a reference list for the person in the centre.
2. Or you can use fruit, flowers, numbers or letters of the alphabet. There should be no duplication.

exchange places as fast as they can. The 'caller' will try to sit in a seat vacated by one or other of them. If he succeeds, the person left standing is the next person to call out two vegetables. The caller also has the choice of calling out *'Salad'*, in which case everyone must change places.

Discussion topics – While the players are catching their breath, and before the next exercise, a light-hearted discussion could be started about why individuals chose to be represented by their particular vegetable.

Your variations

Allow 5–10 minutes
Group size: 8 adults/6 children

Getting acquainted with rhythm (warm-up)

This is a *theatre game* designed to assist group members to learn each other's names, improve concentration, coordination and sense of rhythm.

Recommended for these problems

Model of Human Occupation

Vol. – loss of internal locus of control as indicated by lack of interaction with the environment

Perf. – impairment of interpersonal/communication as indicated by social isolation

– decreased concentration (5 minutes or less)

– loss of vocabulary, e.g. aphasia

– slowing of perceptual-motor skills

Life-style Performance Model

Sens/mo. – slowed sensory-motor output

– aphasia

Cog. – short attention span

Psyc. – difficulty sustaining contact with external stimuli

Intp. – limited social interaction

Stage of group development

This exercise is good for an incohesive group in which the participants do not know each other's names and show mutual lack of interest.[1]

Synopsis

This is an exercise consisting of a clapped rhythm coordinated with the calling of a person's name.

Materials and equipment

Name tags.
A comfortable carpeted room or cushions to sit on.

Procedure

Ask the group members to kneel on the floor in a circle and then in turn to introduce themselves by name.	The circle formation means that each person is within the vision of every other person.
Demonstrate the rhythm as you give the instructions.	To make the exercise easier to learn.

1. It is a useful introductory exercise to use when new members join a group.

Start by giving the following instructions:
'We will learn the rhythm first. To the count of six
and using both hands...
Slap your knees, twice (*one, two*)
Clap your hands together, twice (*three, four*)
Snap your fingers, once with the right hand and
once with the left hand (*five, six*).'

This requires concentration, coordination and a
sense of rhythm.

'We shall repeat the sequence from the beginning
many times, trying to maintain an even pace.'

This will help those whose concentration and
immediate recall is rather poor.

Continue practising until everyone can remember
the actions and do them in time with one another.
(The speed must be relative to that of the slowest
person.)

To reinforce the learning and promote a sense of
individual and group achievement along with
social interaction.

'Now we have learned the actions, at the same
time as everyone snaps their fingers, one player
will call out his own name twice.'

This part of the exercise can be used to
encourage each person to speak up loudly and
distinctly.

'We must all help to keep the rhythm going and...

Encourage the group members to be supportive
of the caller, so that if he becomes muddled he
can join in with the rhythm again.

---

while everyone snaps their fingers again, the
same player will call out the name of another
person twice.'

Using a person's name necessitates recognizing
that person and making eye-contact with him.

'The named person then takes over, firstly calling
his own name twice and then that of yet another
person (always in time to the finger snapping part
of the rhythm), and so on.'[2, 3]

The repetitive nature of the game should assist
everyone to learn and remember each other's
names.

Immediately following the exercise or towards
the end of the session discussion could be
introduced on personal rhythms and how they
manifest themselves in our lives.

Discussion topics   – Was it difficult to keep the clapping rhythm going?
– Do people have different personal rhythms?
– Consider yourself – do you do things fast or slowly?
– In what different ways can people demonstrate their rhythm?
– Do we choose friends with similar rhythms to ourselves?
– Is it possible to adapt one's rhythm and in what circumstances
would it be appropriate?

Your variations

---

2. As practice tends to make the participants more proficient, this exercise can also
be successfully used on a regular basis.
3. The exercise is contraindicated for overactive patients as it is too stimulating.

Allow 1 hour
Group size: 8 adults/6 children

Introductions

This exercise offers an opportunity to practise asking and answering social questions and then sharing what one has learned with a group of people.

Recommended for these problems

Model of Human Occupation

Vol.   – decreased belief in self as indicated by:
         low self-esteem
         hopelessness

Perf.   – impairment of interpersonal communication skills as indicated by:
         social isolation
         limited conversation skills

Life-style Performance Model

Psyc.   – loss of self-esteem

Intp.   – limited social interaction
         – withdrawal from reciprocal interpersonal relationships
         – limited conversation skills

Stage of group development

This is an ideal exercise for a group containing several new members, or for one in which the participants are particularly isolated and withdrawn.

Synopsis

The group divides up into pairs and each pair becomes acquainted with one another through asking and answering questions. Then, each person introduces his partner to the remainder of the group.

Materials and equipment

Paper and pencils.
A comfortable room where simultaneous conversations can be carried on without conflicting with each other.

Procedure

Explain the exercise as follows: 'In order to get to know one another better, we are going to take turns to introduce someone to the group.'	The purpose of the exercise is explained in order to allay the fear of the unknown often held by new members.
'The person on your right will be your partner.'[1]	To eliminate some of the awkwardness in initial conversation.

---

1. If the group members are quite self-assured, suggest that they choose the person they know least, but whom they would like to get to know, as a partner.

At this point it may be appropriate to ask group members what sort of questions are appropriate to ask and answer in this type of social situation.	To develop an awareness of the level of confidentiality that is appropriate at a first meeting.
Invite a group member to write a list of the suggestions and post it up.	To provide a handy reference for those whose concentration is poor.
'Move to a quiet spot in the room and say to each other, "Tell me all about yourself." Collect as much information about one another as you can. In ten minutes, we will reform into a large group.'	The competitive element in this exercise stimulates dialogue and encourages interest in the other person. The time limit gives a work-oriented approach to the exercise.
In ten minutes say, 'Your ten minutes are up. Please move into a large circle.'	To unite physically and thereby recreate some cohesion in the group.
When everyone is seated, ask, 'Who would like to begin to introduce his partner by name and by description?'	To give an an opportunity for an individual to be assertive. Hearing oneself described often increases self-esteem, as details are given that one would normally withold out of modesty.

Continue encouraging each person to take his turn when he feels ready to do so.

Discussion topics
– What feelings did each person experience while doing the exercise?
– Within each pair, how did the conversation go, i.e. did both participate equally, or one more than the other?
– What social situations do you find yourself in where this type of conversation would be both appropriate and necessary?
– If you ask questions that are too personal when you first meet someone what may be the consequences and why?

Your variations

Likes and dislikes

Allow 1 hour
Group size: 8 adults/6 children

This is an exercise in self-awareness and social conversation.

Recommended for these problems	**Model of Human Occupation**	
	Vol.	– inability to make decisions
		– decreased belief in self as indicated by difficulty talking in a group situation
		– limited self-concept
		– diminished sense of personal effectiveness
		– difficulty describing interests
	Perf.	– impairment of interpersonal communication skills as indicated by social isolation
	Life-style Performance Model	
	Psyc.	– ambivalence
		– lowered ability to assess personal skills
		– loss of self-reliance
	Intp.	– limited skills in verbal group interaction
		– limited social interaction

Stage of group development   This is an exercise which enables an unfamiliar, incohesive group to get to know one another and begin to interact.

Synopsis   It requires that each person list the five things they like most and the five things they dislike most on opposite sides of a piece of paper. This information is then used as a basis for discussion.

Materials and equipment   Sheets of paper.
Pencils.
Erasers.
Room with a table and chairs.

Procedure

Invite the group members to sit around the table.	To promote a sense of security and purpose (the solid table ensures a definite distance between the people).
Ask them to pass around the pencils and sheets of paper, keeping one of each for themselves.	To encourage a decision on the part of each person to participate actively.

Then give the following instructions:
'Label one side of your piece of paper with the word *Likes*. Then turn it over and label the other side with the word *Dislikes*.'

'Under the headings write the five things you like most and the five you dislike most.'[1]	To encourage self-awareness through the process of evaluation and discrimination. The lists compiled are usually factual and may relate to recent events in each person's life.
'You have 10 minutes in which to do this.'	To provide a time limit within which to work and encourage each person to apply himself to the task.
'After 10 minutes the sheets of paper will be redistributed amongst the group so that no one has his own.'[2]	This allows the shy person to describe himself through someone else.
'Each person will have an opportunity to read out what is written on the sheet of paper he holds, so that the group can try to guess who wrote it and discuss the contents.'[3]	To promote increased awareness of each other as interesting and unique individuals. To encourage verabal expression and interaction. The puzzle elements make the exercise more stimulating.

Your variations

1. There are many possible variations. The following are just a few examples: *Things you like doing, things you dislike doing* (to assist awareness of how the person spends his time); *Ways in which you behave towards other people, which they like or dislike* (to aid self-awareness and evaluation of the effect of one's behaviour upon others); *Identify problems that you have and list possible ways of dealing with them* (to encourage objectivity and realistic constructive thought). Role-play some of the alternatives to provide an opportunity for the person to experience and/or practise some of his ideas, as well as receive feedback on the solutions.
2. The lists could be put in a hat and each person asked to choose one as he takes his turn. This variation is useful when there are distractable, anxious people in the group who would be reading the list given them rather than listening to the discussion.
3. Where problems, feelings or aspects of behaviour are being identified, it is important that the discussion include constructive alternatives contributed either by the group members, the therapist or, more usefully, by the individual himself.

Name recall
(warm-up)

This is a *theatre game* which improves social interaction, concentration and short-term memory.[1]

Recommended for these problems

Model of Human Occupation
Vol.   – difficulty initiating conversation
Hab.   – loss of valued roles
Perf.   – decreased concentration as indicated by forgetfulness
Life-style Performance Model
Cog.   – short attention span
           – diminished retention and recall
Intp.   – limited ability to initiate conversation

Stage of group development

It is a good exercise to use when working with a group which contains several new members.

Synopsis

Each person introduces himself by name to the group and then shares something personal. He then tries to remember the names and personal contributions of all the people preceding him.

Materials and equipment

None.
Use a room large enough for everyone to sit in a circle and be comfortable.

Procedure

Invite the group members to sit in a circle. Explain the exercise as follows:
'We are going to start today with a theatre game to help improve our concentration and memory. It will give us a chance to practise the art of introducing ourselves to another person and will help the new members learn our names.'

An explanation of the purpose of the exercise may help to allay any anxiety the participants feel.

---

1. The exercise is also suitable for *videotaping*. Watching the replay will provide each person with an opportunity to look at himself and his own behaviour more objectively. Specifically, the tape will show any habits participants have which make communication difficult or impossible (avoiding eye-contact, mumbling, speaking very softly, not paying attention, etc.). Once the habits have been identified each person is in a position to start learning more appropriate and effective ones.

'One person begins by introducing himself to the person on his left, saying, "Hi, my name is ...". He then tells that person something about himself.'[2]

This encourages a person to make specific contact with another person, and gives an opportunity for them to begin learning something about each other.

'The person he is addressing then repeats what he has heard, and turning to the person on *his* left, introduces himself and gives a personal fact. And so it continues around the circle until the last person, who must recite all the names and facts, tells them to the person who started.'

'If one of us cannot remember either a name or fact the game will start again at the beginning.[3] The game is finished when everyone has had his turn.'

This is so that the person who has difficulty remembering has another opportunity to learn the names by repetition.

To start this exercise the therapist may either ask for a *volunteer* or designate someone, bearing in mind that since the game is a progressive one the last person to play has to remember considerably more than the first.[4]

Discussion topics[5] – What does it feel like to be in a room full of strangers?
– Why is it important to remember a person's name?
– Discuss the importance of being able to share personal facts when talking to another person.
– Discuss the importance of paying attention to a person's replies if one is interested in continuing the conversation.

Your variations

2. Initially invite group members to simply share their names. Once these have been learned, they can share superficial facts about themselves, such as 'What is their favourite kind of food?' or 'What do they like doing most in their spare time?' If the group members know one another well then this exercise is an excellent way to help them start sharing facts of a more personal and insightful nature, such as 'What problem brings you to this group?'
3. Go back to the person who started and play the game exactly as before with each person sharing the same personal fact.
4. cf. *Magic box*, p. 117.
5. Since this game is primarily a warm-up technique it is likely that discussion will not follow it immediately, but after other exercises have been used.

Names (warm-up)

Allow 20 minutes
Group size: 10 adults/6 children

This is a *warm-up* exercise. It stimulates group members to be physically active and helps them get to know each other better.

Recommended for these problems

Model of Human Occupation
Vol.   – loss of sense of identity
Perf. – decreased social involvement resulting in social isolation
       – difficulty initiating social interaction
       – slowing of perceptual-motor skills

Life-style Performance Model
Sens/mo. – slowed sensory-motor output
Intp.   – limited social interaction
         – limited ability to initiate conversation

Stage of group development

This is an excellent exercise to use with a group of people who do not know one another.

Synopsis

Each person identifies himself on a name tag. The object of the game is to be the first person to record on paper everyone else's name.

Materials and equipment

Pencils.
Name tags.
Pins.
Sheets of paper.
A spacious room.

Procedure

Explain the exercise as follows:
'Write your name [or occupation, leisure interest, or other variation] on the tag.'[1]

'Pin the tag to the back of your sleeve.

With the name tag in this position the person has to move about in order to avoid being identified.

---

1. Instead of a person's name you could ask group members to put a personal quality on the tag that distinguishes them from others, e.g. occupation, leisure interests or a famous person they would like to be.

When I say "start," move around, read and write down all the names you can see.'

This encourages (1) an increased awareness of his position in relation to those around him, and (2) defensive tactics as he attempts to trick others into revealing their identity.

'The first person to collect all the names (the number in the group) is the winner.'

When three or more people have completed their lists, reform as a group and ask each person to identify himself.

To satisfy the curiosity of those who had not finished and to match names with faces.

Discussion topics
- The difficulty remembering people's names when you first meet them.
- If one of the variations has been chosen, discussion can be about choices made by each person.

Your variations

Pass the ball
(warm-up)

Allow 5–10 minutes or 1 hour
Group size: 12 adults/6 children

This is primarily a *warm-up* technique to provide personal introductions, assist name-learning and promote communication between participants.[1]

Recommended for these problems

Model of Human Occupation
Perf. — slowing of perceptual motor skills
— difficulty initiating social interaction
— decreased social involvement
— impairment of interpersonal skills

Life-style Performance Model
Sens/mo. — slowed sensory-motor output
Intp. — withdrawal from reciprocal interpersonal relationships
— limited social interaction
— limited ability to initiate conversation

Stage of group development

This is an excellent exercise to use as a *warm-up* for a group of people who are particularly quiet or withdrawn and do not know one another.

Synopsis

One person in the group passes the ball to another person and at the same time offers some verbal information about himself to the recipient.

Materials and equipment

A ball (choose a large, light one if possible).
Chairs (if the participants are unable to sit on the floor).

Procedure

Invite the group members to sit down in as small a circle as possible.	This tends to provide physical closeness between group members and makes passing the ball across the circle easier.

1. This exercise is suitable for *videotaping*. The replay can be used to show participants how they converse with one another and, more specifically, to identify potential communication problems (e.g. avoiding eye-contact, talking very softly, answering questions in a vague or indirect way, reluctance to share personal information, etc.). If problems are identified, these can form the basis for a discussion.

Place the ball in the centre of the circle and explain the exercise as follows:

'One person in the group will pick up the ball and give it to another person saying: "My name is ..." The recipient, in turn, will give the ball to a third person saying. "My name is ..." and so on.'[2,3]

This involves the simultaneous actions of making physical contact with a chosen person and introducing oneself to him. Eye-contact and clear diction are encouraged.

'If, at any time, you do not wish to participate, then place the ball back in the centre of the circle.'

This provides an opportunity for opting out and the decision to do so is expressed nonverbally.

'Anyone else may pick up the ball and continue with the exercise.'

'When everyone has said their names several times, the sentence will be extended to include the recipient's name, i.e. "My name is ..., your name is ...", each time you pass the ball on.'

This improves the skills of recognition and recall. The associated physical contact acts as an added stimulus for those whose attention span and/or contact with reality is poor.

'Now that you have learned everyone's name, when you pass the ball on, tell the recipient something about yourself, prefixing your statement with his name.'[4]

This encourages the participants to share information about themselves.

The exercise can be progressed stage by stage to include such topics as, 'Now tell the recipient how you are feeling today.'[5,6]

This encourages the identification and expression of feelings in a direct and specific manner.

The exercise could be concluded in the following manner:

'Finally, you can ask the recipient of your ball a question. He may answer you and then he can turn to another person with a question.'

This promotes conversational exchanges between people but in a very structured way. It encourages the use of initiative and an awareness of other people.

---

2. To provide an outlet for restlessness, ask the participants to walk across the circle and give the ball to the person they have chosen.
3. To stimulate the motor senses (e.g. reflexes, muscle coordination and control) rather than intimate interpersonal contact, ask the participants to stand up and either throw or bounce the ball to one another when they speak.
4. By sharing information in this way, new members joining a group are provided with some cues for further conversation.
5. In a smaller group members will get to know and trust one another more quickly than in a larger group.
6. As therapist you can decide what information will be helpful for the players to share with one another. Suggestions can also be elicited from the group members themselves.

Discussion topics
- Why is it important to be able to share information about ourselves with other people?
- In what situations must one be able to talk to other people and why?
- Why is it sometimes difficult to talk directly to another person?
- What nonverbal behaviours do people sometimes do in order to avoid talking to others?

Your variations

Allow 10–30 minutes
Group size: 10 adults/6 children

The matchbox is ...?
(warm-up)

This is an exercise to develop the capacity to be observant and use words that are descriptive.

Recommended for these problems

Model of Human Occupation

Vol.
- decreased belief in self as indicated by difficulty talking in a group situation
- loss of internal locus of control as indicated by lack of interaction with the environment

Perf.
- neurological deficiencies as indicated by visual-motor deficits

Life-style Performance Model

Sens/mo.
- decreased visual/tactile discrimination

Psyc.
- difficulty sustaining contact with external stimuli

Intp.
- limited skills in verbal group interaction

Stage of group development

This exercise could be used with a group of very withdrawn patients to help them to stay in touch with their immediate situation and begin to communicate. If the exercise is used in this way the time allowance should be extended until the level of participation indicates that progression to another exercise is appropriate.

Synopsis

An article is passed around and as each person receives it he is invited to contribute one thing towards its description.

Materials and equipment

Small objects, such as pencil, ashtray, key, vase, jar, etc.
Use a small familiar room.

Procedure

Invite the group members to sit in a circle.

Explain the exercise as follows:
'I am going to pass a small *article*, (e.g. a matchbox) around the group.'[1]

---

1. These articles can be collected beforehand or each person can be asked to produce something he has on him at the time.

'When each person receives it, he is invited to describe something about the *article*[2] before passing it on to the next person.'	To improve observation and tactile discrimination skills. The process of passing the object encourages nonverbal interaction.
'The object of the game is to describe as many aspects of the *article* as we can without repetition.'	To encourage greater concentration and originality.
Continue passing the same *article* around until all possibilities have been exhausted and then invite a group member to introduce a new *article*.	This stimulates the generation of a wide variety of observations, necessitating some creative thinking.
Group members can be invited to make personal contributions.	Producing personal items may encourage a greater degree of interest and participation.

Your variations

2. With patients whose thought processes are very slow it is sometimes advisable to stimulate ideas by suggestion (e.g. as to shape, size, smell, texture, weight and use). This may be done as you give the instructions or may need to be given as coaching to each person in turn.

This is my life

Allow 1 hour
Group size: 8 adults/6 children

(Adapted from Stalker.[1])

This is an exercise to enable a person identify and talk about important aspects of their life through an art activity.

Recommended for these problems

Model of Human Occupation

Vol.
- limited self-concept
- difficulty describing interests

Perf.
- impairment of interpersonal communication skills as indicated by:
  - social isolation
  - limited conversation skills
  - deficient paralinguistic skills

Life-style Performance Model

Psyc.
- loss of self-esteem

Intp.
- limited social interaction
- withdrawal from reciprocal interpersonal relationships
- limited conversation skills
- poor paralinguistic skills

Stage of group development

This is a useful exercise to do with a group that is meeting for the first time or is in the beginning stages of developing group identity and cohesion.

Synopsis

Each person is asked to draw eight simple pictures of people or things which represent different aspects of their lives. They then talk about the resulting poster.

Materials and equipment

Large sheets of paper. Coloured construction paper can be used for children.
Felt pens, wax crayons or pencils.
Use a room with a large table and chairs.

Procedure

Ask everyone to sit around the table ...	To promote a sense of group cohesion and a purposeful atmosphere.
and help themselves to a piece of paper and felt pen.	This allows each person to make a physical decision to participate.

The remaining felt pens, etc. can be placed in the middle of the table.	To encourage cooperative interaction while working.
Explain the exercise as follows: 'Today we are going to do an art project that will help you identify the people and things that are especially important to you in your life.' 'At the top of your piece of paper write. "This is my life".'	
'Then draw a line from top to bottom dividing the paper in half.'	Demonstrate if need be.
'Once you have done that, then draw three lines from left to right so you will end up with eight boxes.	You may wish to show an example to assist those group members who have trouble following verbal directions.
Enquire if anyone needs more time.	
Once everyone is ready say: 'Take some time to think about your life and particularly the important people in it. Can anyone think of an example?	Asking group members to contribute ideas encourages them to begin thinking in a general way.
Be ready with some suggestions if ideas are not forthcoming, e.g. immediate family, relatives, friends, boss, pets, etc.	
Continue: 'Now consider the things you enjoy doing. These could be activities you actually do or would like to do.' Again as leader you should be ready with some suggestions, e.g. sports, hobbies, etc. 'Other ideas you can think of could include where you were born, your favourite movie, flavour of ice-cream, special talent, etc.'	
'Make a simple drawing or use words in each of the eight squares to represent different aspects of your life.'	To encourage each person to identify a variety of supportive people, interests, etc.
'At the bottom of the page you may wish to write a personal "motto", which is a short sentence or phrase that sums up a personal belief or course of action, e.g. the early bird catches the worm.'	

When most people have finished ask: 'Does anyone need more time?'	To give those who are not ready the responsibility for informing the group that they need more time.
When everyone has completed the exercise, invite each person to share what is on their poster with the group.	This provides an excellent opportunity to develop awareness of what is appropriate information to share with others when you are getting to know them. The nonverbal skills of making eye-contact, using facial expression and speaking clearly are encouraged.
Encourage group members to ask questions.	To practise the art of asking appropriate questions in a social situation.

Discussion topics
  – Was the project easy or difficult? Why?
  – What topics and personal information are suitable to share with someone who you have just met? Why?
  – What topics and personal information are not suitable to share with someone who you have just met? Why?
  – Did you choose a motto? What does it say about you?

Your variations

REFERENCES

1. Stalker, A. (1991) *Bridges to Competence, Activities for Theme-based Social Skills Groups.* Available from the Occupational Therapy Department, British Columbia's Children's Hospital, 4480 Oak St., Vancouver, B.C., V6H 3V4, Canada.

Who stole the cookie from the cookie jar?

(warm-up)

Allow 5–10 minutes
Group size: 12 adults/6 children

This exercise is a *theatre game* which uses rhythm to improve coordination and concentration.

Recommended for these problems

Model of Human Occupation
Perf. – decreased concentration (5–15 minutes)
– slowing of perceptual-motor skills
– impairment of interpersonal/communication skills as indicated by social isolation

Life-style Performance Model
Sens/mo. – slowed sensory-motor output
Cog. – short attention span
Intp. – limited social interaction

Stage of group development
The exercise can be used successfully with most groups.

Synopsis
This is an exercise in which words are said in time to a clapped rhythm.

Materials and equipment
Blackboard and chalk.
Use a room that is spacious.

Procedure

Before the session starts, write the words to be spoken on the blackboard. Words to be written up: 'Who stole the cookie from the cookie jar?' 'Was it you number…?' 'Who me?' 'Yes, you.' 'Couldn't be.' 'Then who?' 'Number …'	This is to assist anyone who has difficulty remembering them due to short attention span.
Invite the players to kneel on the floor in a circle … and to number off to the right. The leader is usually Number One.[1]	A circle enables everyone to see everyone else and promotes a sense of cohesion. Encourage the players to speak up clearly, so that everyone can hear.

---

1. If the players are familiar with the exercise the leader can be a group member.

Explain the game as follows:
'The leader claps his hands in a simple rhythm which the rest of us imitate.' (Begin with a very slow and simple rhythm so that the speed of it can be increased later on in the game.)

This requires concentration, motor coordination and a sense of rhythm.

'Then when everyone is familiar with the rhythm the leader begins speaking in time to it, saying…

Leader: "Who stole the cookie from the cookie jar? Was it you Number Four?"' (Any number from amongst the group members may be used).

The exercise becomes more difficult at this point, demanding greater concentration and psychomotor coordination.

'*Number Four*: "Who me?"
Leader: "Yes, you."
Number Four: "Couldn't be."
Leader: "Then who?"
Number Four: "Number Ten."'

This provides an opportunity to practise quick verbal interaction.

Since the players do not know which one of them will be called next they need to remain alert.

'*Number Ten*: "Who me?"
Number Four: "Yes, you"
Number Ten: "Couldn't be."
…and so on.'

If at any point one of the players fails to speak in time to the rhythm the game stops, and starts again with this particular person as the new leader.

The person who is finding the exercise difficult assumes a more influential position in the group…

He begins his own rhythm and then in time to it says, "Who stole the cookie from the cookie jar?" … and so on

That allows him to set a slower pace for those with slowed sensory–motor output.

As the players become proficient, the speed of the rhythm can be increased.

This will have the effect of intensifying the need to concentrate and react quickly.

Your variations

Word circle (warm-up)

Allow 15–30 minutes
Group size: 10 adults/6 children

This is an exercise to improve a person's ability to think and speak clearly, especially when he is surprised.

Recommended for these problems

Model of Human Occupation
Vol. – decreased expectations of success
Perf. – difficulty speaking voluntarily due to decrease in sponta-neous psychomotor behaviour
– difficulty thinking quickly due to deficiencies in process skills
– decreased concentration (5 minutes or less)

Life-style Performance Model
Sens/mo. – difficulty speaking clearly
Cog. – slowness of thought -processing
– short attention span
Intp. – limited spontaneous conversation

Stage of group development

This is an appropriate exercise for a rather apathetic group of patients who will not or cannot do a physically active exercise.[1]

Synopsis

The exercise takes the form of a game in which each player calls out a set number of words all beginning with the same letter, in a limited period of time.

Materials and equipment

A small object, e.g. book, bean bag, ball.
Small carpeted room.

Procedure

Instruct the players to sit on the floor in as small a circle as possible.	This encourages close association with another person and gives a sense of unity to the group.
Explain the rules of the game as follows: 'The leader of this game sits in the centre of the circle while an object is being passed around from player to player at an even speed.'	Sitting in the centre of the circle makes the leader an integral part of the whole group. Passing the object helps each person to concentrate and remain involved.

1. This is an excellent game and the authors recommend that it is played frequently as proficiency increases with practice.

'The leader closes his eyes and claps his hands once.
He then announces a letter of the alphabet, excluding X and Z.'

Two decisions are involved here, when to clap and what letter to call. The leader is also required to speak out clearly.

'When he claps, the person in the group to touch the object last calls out a predetermined number of words (these can be nouns, verbs, adjectives, adverbs, etc.) beginning with the announced letter.'

This encourages fluency in both thinking and speaking. The skills of concentration, retention and recall are used, as well as the ability to select appropriate words. Increased vocabulary may also result.

The number of words required should be small at first and increased as the players become more proficient.

Achieving success in calling the words will improve a person's confidence and decrease his anxiety about failing. This will ultimately enable him to become proficient.

'Meanwhile the object is still being passed around the circle and if the caller fails to list off the required number of words before the object returns to him he replaces the leader in the centre of the circle.'

This imposes a time limit in which to complete the task and enables the person to experience a situation requiring quick thinking. If a person fails to think of the correct number of words he changes his role from that of player to leader.

'If the caller succeeds then he remains in his place and the game continues with the original leader.'[2,3]

Your variations

---

2. To encourage a sense of responsibility, invite the group as a whole to see that the rules of the game are adhered to. They should also decide on the number of words to be called at any one time (bearing in mind that this number be low enough to provide a sense of achievement and high enough to be challenging).
3. Variations may include: words that rhyme or words in a particular category (e.g. countries, animals).

Comment cards

Allow 45 minutes
Group size: 10 adults/6 children

This exercise is designed to increase an individual's awareness of other people, while involving him in a social situation which is not stressful.

Recommended for these problems

Model of Human Occupation
Vol. – decreased belief in self as indicated by low self-esteem
– lack of interest in others
Perf. – impairment of interpersonal communication skills as indicated by social isolation
– slowing of perceptual-motor skills
Life-style Performance Model
Sens/mo. – slowed sensory-motor output
Intp. – decreased interest in others
– limited social interaction
Psyc. – loss of self-esteem

Stage of group development

This exercise is suitable for a group in which the members are only superficially familiar with one another. It is a useful exercise for the development of group cohesion and can be used as a precursor to 'Compliments'.

Synopsis

Each person thinks of a word or phrase to describe each member of the group. He writes his comment on a card which has been taped to the member's back and the descriptions are then shared and discussed.

Materials and equipment

8 cm × 13 cm cards.
Masking tape.
Pens.
Use a room with chairs.

Procedure

Explain the exercise as follows:
'This exercise helps you discover how you appear to other people.'

By pointing out the personal gain achieved through the exercise, the leader can more effectively gain the attention and cooperation of those individuals who have difficulty participating in group therapy.

Ask some members to help you hand out pens and cards, and ask them to assist in taping cards to people's backs.

To encourage active participation by those with limited social interaction or low self-esteem.

'We are going to move about the room. As you pass each person, think of a word or phrase which you consider aptly describes them and…

Physically moving torwards and among other people is helpful for those members handicapped by feelings of social isolation.

then write it on the card on their back.'

This encourages those with limited communication skills to say say positive things to others anonymously.

When each member's card has a comment from everyone, ask the group to reform into a circle. Then invite each person to read out his list of comments.

Discussion   – Encourage each person to discuss his feelings about the comments he received; then assist the discussion to develop into a view of how he feels about himself.

Your variations

Continuing story

Allow 10–30 minutes
Group size: 8 adults/6 children

This is a *theatre game* to help individuals feel more confident speaking to a group of people, without any preparation.[1]

Recommended for these problems

Model of Human Occupation

Vol.   – diminished sense of personal effectiveness
Perf.   – decrease in spontaneous psychomotor behaviour as indicated by difficulty speaking spontaneously
           – decreased concentration (5–15 minutes)
           – difficulty formulating ideas

Life-style Performance Model

Sens/mo. – limited spontaneous conversation
Cog.   – short attention span
           – loss of ability to generate ideas
Psyc.   – loss of self-reliance

Stage of group development

This exercise is best used in a group that has developed some unity and where the members are actively participating to the best of their abilities.

Synopsis

A continuing story is told by the group members. Each person speaks in turn adding on to the previous speaker's words until a logical conclusion is reached.

Materials and equipment

None.
Use a familiar room.

---

1. The exercise can be *videotaped*. The replay can be watched for fun or to look more specifically at some of the difficulties participants encountered. These might be such things as not being able to think of anything to say, difficulty paying attention and not speaking audibly. Look for nonverbal communication strengths and weaknesses such as making eye-contact appropriately, use of body posture and gestures to enhance the story telling.

Procedure

Invite from four to seven players to form a line...[2]	This provides an opportunity for volunteers to come forward.[3]
in front of the audience... and one person from the audience to be the *Director*.[4]	To promote a sense of theatre. This provides an opportunity for someone to try out a position of leadership.
Explain the exercise as follows: 'The audience chooses a *hero* about whom the players are going to tell a story.'	This encourages audience participation.
The *Director* then says: 'The *hero* of your story is ...' and points to one of the players, who immediately begins to make up a story about the designated hero.	This person is encouraged to speak spontaneously.
The player continues with his story until the *Director* points to a different player (the game is more entertaining if the switch occurs while the person speaking is in the middle of a sentence).	
This person takes the story up where the previous speaker left off and so the game continues.	
'The only rules are that the story must be grammatically correct and coherent.'	This means that the players need to listen very carefully as well as concentrate upon the *Director*.
'It is the responsibility of the audience to edit the story, that is, to listen for any grammatical mistakes, repeated words, etc. and as soon as they hear one to shout "error".'	The continuous audience participation in this way requires concentration and active involvement in the game.
At this point the story stops, while the player who made the error joins the audience.	

2. Since this exercise is dependent upon there being enough people to be both *story tellers* and *audience*, the number of *story tellers* should be no more than half the group.
3. Depending on the degree of response to the therapist's request for volunteers, the therapist may need to encourage or even choose *story tellers*.
4. Initially it may be advisable for the therapist to take the role of *Director*, thereby demonstrating how to direct the game and promote enjoyment. A withdrawn person might be encouraged to participate as the *Director's assistant* and select the speakers.

'The *Director*, who must remember the last word that was spoken, repeats it and points to another player and the story continues until one player is left.'

To refresh the players' memories for those with short attention span.

'This person concludes the story with a moral and is applauded.'

The game continues with a new set of players and a new *hero*.

Invite discussion at the end.

Discussion topics
– Discuss any feelings that were evoked by having to speak up in front of a group.
– Discuss the effect of audience participation, laughter and applause upon the story-tellers.

Your variations

Geography (warm-up)

Allow 10 minutes (minimum)
Group size: 10 adults/6 children

This is a *warm-up* technique. It is an exercise which assists a person to think quickly, to concentrate and to practise immediate recall.

Recommended for these problems

Model of Human Occupation

Vol.	– decreased belief in self as indicated by loss of self-esteem
Perf.	– decreased concentration (5 minutes or less)
	– deficiency in process skills as indicated by difficulty thinking quickly

Life-style Performance Model

Cog.	– short attention span
	– diminished retention and recall
	– slowness in thought-processing
Psyc.	– loss of self-esteem

Stage of group development

A group that is meeting for the first time can attain some degree of cohesion from this exercise. However, it is also enjoyable and useful to do with a group at any stage of its development.

Synopsis

Each person in turn says the name of a geographical place. The name he chooses must begin with the last letter of the geographical name that his predecessor chose.[1]

Materials and equipment

Use a room with chairs or a carpeted floor.

Procedure

Invite the group members to sit in a circle.	To unite the group physically.
Explain the exercise as follows: 'The game begins with one person saying the name of a place (e.g. *London*). The person seated to his left will then give another geographical name beginning with the last letter of the previous word (if we follow the example, then the place name must begin with *N*, e.g. *New York*) and so the game continues around the circle.'	In order to take his turn, each player must concentrate on what the previous player says and assimilate what he has heard. This will improve his ability to retain and recall information.

1. The exercise is contraindicated for a group containing excessively active patients, or for patients for whom recall is so difficult that participating would be ego-deflating. People who do not speak English well can achieve success at this game, as they are not limited to English names only.

'No names may be repeated.'	This means that as the game progresses more and more names have to be remembered.
'However, if a person cannot think of a name, anyone may give him a clue in the form of a question (e.g. "What is the largest city in the USA?" Then he will remember *New York*).'	It is important, therefore, to encourage helpful communication between the group members and provide an opportunity (within the rules) for the restless person to participate when it is not his turn.
Change to another exercise when you see signs of the first person becoming restless.	Since this is a *warm-up* activity, it is best to stop while everyone is still interested and participating actively.

Your variations

Allow 5–10 minutes per pair
Group size: 12 adults/6 children

Hand puppets

This is a *theatre game* that helps a person talk easily and with more confidence in a group situation. It may also stimulate a greater awareness of one of the nonverbal aspects of communication, i.e. hand gestures.[1]

Recommended for these problems

Model of Human Occupation

Vol.   – decreased belief in self as indicated by difficulty talking in a group situation
Hab.   – feelings of incompetence
Perf.   – deficiencies in process skills as indicated by difficulty thinking quickly
– slowing of perceptual-motor skills

Life-style Performance Model

Sens/mo.   – slowed sensory motor output
Cog.   – slowness in thought-processing
Intp.   – limited skills in verbal group interaction

Stage of group development

This exercise is most successful with a group in which the participants are fairly comfortable with each other.

Synopsis

In this exercise two people stand, one behind the other,[2] before an audience (made up of the rest of the group). The front person delivers a short speech, while the back person, placing his arms forward so that they appear to belong to his partner, uses his hands to augment what is being said.

Materials and equipment

None
Use a familiar and preferably carpeted room.

---

1. The exercise is suitable for *videotaping*. The replay will be fun to watch and will enable the participants to look carefully at such speaking skills as: being able to talk loudly; being able to talk at a reasonable pace; and being able to talk in an interesting manner. The replay will show if each person was able to organize and express his thoughts clearly. It will also illustrate the importance of hand gestures and the part they play in communication.
2. If physical proximity is too stressful or not possible, side-by-side miming is an alternative.

Procedure

Invite the players to sit on the floor in a group.	This brings everyone together as a cohesive unit to form the audience.
Ask if there are two volunteers of about the same height, who are willing to stand up before the audience, one (*B*) behind the other (*A*).[3]	It is important to provide an opportunity for each person to make the decision about whether he wishes to participate. Working with another person is easier and less frightening than doing it alone.
Explain the exercise as follows: 'The front person holds *B* close to his own body, by clasping his hands behind *B*'s back, and…	Standing very close together will assist them to work more easily as one unit.
'*B* puts his arms forward so that they look as though they belong to the front person' (see illustration).	
'The front person then delivers a short speech to the audience…[4]	Encourage him to talk spontaneously even if it is only for a very short time.

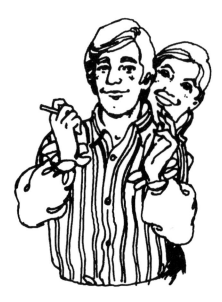

---

3. An alternative is to have one pair of players carrying on a conversation with another pair. As the number of people on *stage* increases so the amount of attention focused on each individual decreases. This may encourage more people to participate.
4. If *A* does not have any ideas the therapist should have a few suggestions prepared (see Suggestions at the end of the exercise).

'and his partner (*B*), using his hands, gesticulates in order to augment what is being said.'	To work as a team, *B* will have to concentrate on what is being said and can participate in the speech using nonverbal skills.
Encourage the audience to participate with laughter, applause, etc.	This is very important as it provides positive support and encouragement for the two players.
'Then, keeping the same positions, the procedure can be reversed, i.e. *B* gesticulates and...	
'*A* makes up a monologue to fit the motions of *B*'s hands.'[5]	In this way *A* is encouraged to speak spontaneously, without being self-conscious.

Suggestions for 'hand puppets'

- A politician giving an election speech.
- A person giving the vote of thanks after a lecture.
- A demonstrator in a store, selling an all-purpose chopping utensil.
- An announcer giving a weather forecast or reading the news.
- Telling a story.
- One person interviewing another who has just climbed the highest mountain in the world, or eaten the most hamburgers.
- Two women having a conversation about some clothes they have purchased.

Your variations

---

5. Stress that the sentences do not have to form a logical story as long as they fit the gestures and actions. This should help to introduce an atmosphere of comedy and enjoyment into the exercise.

Monologue or dialogue

Allow 1 hour
Group size: 12 adults

This is an exercise to illustrate the difference between two types of communication,[1] that is, between a monologue and a dialogue.

Recommended for these problems

Model of Human Occupation
Perf.   – deficiencies in process skills as indicated by difficulty planning
       – difficulty initiating conversation due to loss of interpersonal skills
       – decreased concentration (5–15 minutes)[2]

Life-style Performance Model
Cog.   – short attention span
       – difficulty making choices
Intp.   – limited ability to initiate conversation

Stage of group development

This exercise is excellent for a group in which the members are still unfamiliar with each other. No feeling of group cohesion is needed.[3]

Synopsis

One person is asked to describe a diagram from a drawing. Each person listens and attempts to reproduce the diagram on paper. No questions or gestures are allowed. A second diagram is then described with both questions and gestures. The difference between these two experiences is discussed.

Materials and equipment

Tables.[4]
Chairs.
Diagram cards (see sample diagram ideas at the end of the exercise).[5]
Sheets of paper approximately the same size as the diagram cards, e.g. 8 cm × 13 cm.

---

1. The exercise is suitable for *videotaping*. Afterwards the replay can be used to look at and discuss specific difficulties that the participants experienced in trying to communicate. The tape will also help participants recall how they felt at any one time.
2. Since it is an exercise where all the participants are involved actively all the time it is suitable for patients who have a short attention span and who need constant stimulation if they are to maintain any contact with reality.
3. Patients with temporal lobe lesions are likely to find this exercise very difficult. It is important, therefore, that the therapist makes an accurate assessment of how complex the diagrams should be for the participants to achieve success and yet be stimulated.
4. To promote a sense of responsibility, you can invite the group to prepare the room and materials.
5. To increase self-esteem, invite the participants to design their own diagram cards.

Pencils.
Erasers.
Sharpener.

Procedure

Ask the group members to sit around the table(s)	
Pass around the pencils and sheets of paper inviting each person to take one of each.	This encourages each person to take an active step in participating.
Explain the exercise as follows: 'One person in the group will be given a card on which there is a diagram. Only he may look at it.'	This provides an opportunity to experience planning and leadership.
'He will describe the diagram slowly and as accurately as he can without using gestures...	This encourages succinct, logical description, attention to detail, accurate judgement and concentration. It exercises the ability to perceive a shape and translate that perception into words.
'while the rest of the group attempt to reproduce this diagram on paper from the instructions they hear.'	This exercises the capacity to form a concept from auditory stimuli and reproduce this concept in graphic form. It assists concentration, attention to detail and accurate judgement.
'No one may ask any questions. Try to be aware of any reactions or feelings you may have while doing the task.'	This promotes self-awareness, especially related to feelings in a situation where the communication is one-way only. The therapist should observe the reactions so that she can use her observations to stimulate discussion.
'On completing the drawing there will be an opportunity for you to discuss your reactions and ascertain how accurate your diagram is before we proceed.'	This provides an opportunity for heightening awareness of the feelings experienced during the task and will focus attention on the problems and/or frustrations inherent in one-way communication.
Ask if there is a volunteer who wants to describe the first diagram and give him the card (if there is no volunteer the therapist takes this role).	This transfers leadership from the therapist to the participants.
When the first part of the exercise has been completed explain the second part as follows: 'Another person will describe a different diagram, this time gestures can be used.'	This provides an opportunity to use gestures to clarify words. This enables more than one person to experience being the leader.

'Again each group member will attempt to reproduce this from the description but this time you may ask questions.'

This will promote two-way communication. The participants will ask questions to clarify points and so experience the feelings that result from successful communication.

'Again try to be aware of your reactions and feelings while doing this exercise.'

This encourages the participants to be more aware of themselves in a particular situation.

When the task is completed to the satisfaction of the group members, invite them to discuss the exercise.

SOME SUGGESTIONS FOR DIAGRAMS

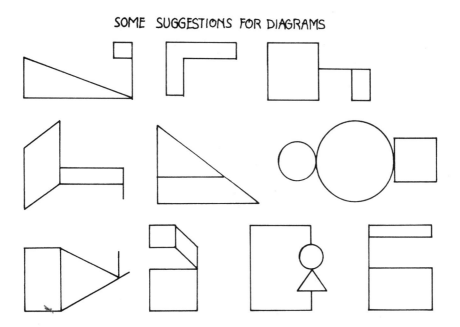

Discussion topics   Compare and contrast the two exercises considering the following:

- What feelings were evoked?
- How important were the gestures in aiding communication?
- How do these experiences (in communication) compare with our daily lives?
- Why is it important to be able to ask questions?
- Are there situations in your daily life which illustrate the two types of communication?

Your variations

Newspaper quiz

Allow 1 hour
Group size: 8 adults/6 children

This is an exercise to stimulate interest in and awareness of current events. It also encourages teamwork.

Recommended for these problems	**Model of Human Occupation**
	Vol. – decreased belief in self as indicated by difficulty talking in a group situation
	– limited awareness of community resources
	– loss of internal locus of control as indicated by lack of interaction with the environment
	Perf. – inability to problem-solve
	Life-style Performance Model
	Cog. – difficulty problem-solving
	– limited skills in community awareness
	Psyc. – difficulty sustaining contact with external stimuli
	Intp. – limited skills in verbal group interaction

Stage of group development   This exercise can be used with a variety of groups but, because of its competitive element, it is particularly useful in fostering group cohesion.

Synopsis   The exercise takes the form of a competitive game in which each team has to hunt through a newspaper for the answer to a specific question.

Materials and equipment   1 complete daily newspaper for each team of 3 to 4 people.
1 table for each team.
Chairs.
Paper.
Pencils.
Blackboard and chalk upon which a visual record of the results can be kept.

Procedure

Beforehand prepare a list of questions, the answers to which will be found in the newspaper (see Suggestions at the at the end of this exercise). Number or label the tables.	To give an opportunity for community awareness.
Invite the group members to form teams of three or four people and sit one team to a table.	To form a team requires making contact with other people through verbal interaction.

Give the following instructions:
'On your table you will find a number which represents your team, a complete copy of today's newspaper and some pencils and paper.[1]

Ask if there are volunteers willing to be the *question-master* or *score-keeper*. The therapist may need to assist the volunteers.	Being *question-master* or *score-keeper* can be a suitable role for someone who feels the exercise is beneath him or for someone who might otherwise remain uninvolved.
'The *question-master* will read out a question and...'	This requires clear, distinct speech.
'the first team to find the correct answer in the newspaper will receive a point.'	To encourage problem solving and cooperative interaction between the members of each team. At this time the therapist can observe how each person participates within his team.
'The *score-keeper* will assign a point to the appropriate team and then the *question-master* will go on to the next question.'	To provide an opportunity for responsibility and cooperation between the teams and the volunteers.
'The winning team will be the one which obtains the highest number of points overall.'[2]	To provide an incentive for maximum effort and participation.

Suggestions for 'Newspaper quiz' questions

– What is today's weather forecast?
– What film is now playing at the *Odeon*?
– Who won the football game last night?
– What store is advertising a Winter Sale?
– Which large building was reported to have burned down last night?
– What problem was Mr Brown writing about in *Letters to the Editor*?
– At what times can you watch a television news bulletin during the evening?
– What is today's horoscope for those born in the beginning of May?
– On what page are *Jobs Available* advertised?
– How much rent is being asked for the one bedroom apartment at 1611 Forge Street?

In preparing the questions consider these points:

1. What information in the newspaper would be of value to this particular group?

---

1. When there are more than two teams competing, it may be advisable that they write their answers down rather than call them out. The answers can be checked at the end of the quiz.
2. With some patients (e.g. children, adolescents, or chronically disabled adults), a prize for the winning team may be the additional stimulus which helps to maintain their interest and involvement.

2. Should you choose information in large print if there are some group members who are on large amounts of medication and have blurred vision?

3. Are the questions difficult enough to be stimulating, yet easy enough to provide a sense of achievement?

4. Do you need to give hints on the location of the answer in the paper?

5. Have you prepared enough questions? (Allow approximately 1 minute per question.)

Your variations

Persuasion

Allow 10–30 minutes
Group size: 8 adults/6 children

This is a *theatre game* involving spontaneous self-expression and social interaction.[1]

Recommended for these problems

Model of Human Occupation

Vol.   – diminished sense of personal effectiveness as indicated by low self-confidence

Perf.   – impairment of interpersonal communication as indicated by social anxiety
       – unassertive in social interaction
       – decrease in psychomotor behaviour as indicated by difficulty speaking voluntarily

Life-style Performance Model

Psyc.   – loss of self-reliance
       – feelings of anxiety

Intp.   – decreased assertiveness in social situations
       – limited spontaneous conversation

Stage of group development

It is recommended that this exercise be done with a group whose members are well enough acquainted that they feel safe to improvise.

Synopsis

A player from the group initiates and develops a skit with an opponent who is seated in a chair. The purpose of the skit is to persuade the opponent to get up from his seat.

Materials and equipment

Chair.
Use a familiar room that is quiet.

Procedure

Invite the players to sit in a large circle on the floor and to find comfortable positions.	To encourage everyone to feel relaxed and thereby, make participation in the exercise easier.
Create a centre stage by placing a chair in the middle of the circle and...	

---

1. The exercise is suitable for *videotaping*. The replay will be fun to watch for all members. The participants will be able to view their abilities to speak spontaneously, to be assertive, or to be persuasive.

ask if there is a volunteer who would like to sit in the chair.	To provide an opportunity for a member to choose to be the centre of attention.
Explain the exercise as follows: 'The object of this game is to persuade the person in the chair to get up from it. You may use any means to achieve this, apart from moving the chair or physical force.'	
'Any player may approach the person in the chair and...'[2]	To encourage spontaneous participation.
'through his actions and/or conversation set the scene.'[3]	To provide an opportunity for self-expression.
'The two of them converse until the seated player is finally persuaded to stand up.'	To assist the formation of a brief relationship with another person and to practise assertive communication with him.
'Other players may join in the conversation at any point if they wish to.'	This freedom allows individuals from the audience to support and encourage the players by spontaneously participating with them.
'Once the seated player does stand up he re-joins the circle. His opponent, taking the seat, waits to be approached by another player who starts a new skit.'	To allow as many players as possible the chance to participate, especially those who are shy or self-conscious and require some encouragement.
As the game continues, encourage the person in the chair to be more reluctant to give up his position.	This will allow the players to be more subtle and skilful in their handling of the situation.
Audience participation should be encouraged at all times (i.e. laughter, applause, verbal encouragement, etc.).	To involve the maximum number of people.

2. Unless the players are very self-confident, it is likely they will hesitate in coming forward initially. Since this is an exercise in spontaneity, we do not suggest that specific people are asked to participate, rather that the leader demonstrates the game using very ordinary familiar scenes (see Suggestions at the end of the exercise). In this way the group members can be encouraged to feel safe enough to act out their own ideas.
3. For example, a player might approach the person in the chair walking like an old man and make a comment that sets the scene of a bus; or he may walk briskly and say, 'Good morning, madam. Is there a particular shoe that interests you?', thereby setting the scene in a shoe shop.

Suggestions for 'Persuasion'   Choose situations which are familiar, easy to enact and naturally require that one of the participants is seated. They should also lend themselves to comedy and improvisation. Some suitable situations might be:

- Watching television.
- Waiting for your appointment in the doctor's office.
- Finding yourself in the wrong seat at the theatre.
- Travelling on the bus.
- Drinking coffee at your local coffee shop.
- Sitting on a park bench enjoying the sunshine during your lunch hour.
- Choosing your desk on the first day of school.

Your variations

Allow 1 hour
Group size: 8 adults/6 children

Save yourself

This is an exercise in public speaking.[1]

Recommended for these problems

Model of Human Occupation

Vol.
– feelings of powerlessness over personal actions
– inhibited self-expression due to decreased expectancy of success

Perf.
– decreased concentration (5–15 minutes)
– deficiencies in processing skills affecting planning
– confused thinking due to neurological deficiencies
– deficiency in paralinguistic skills

Life-style Performance Model

Cog.
– confused thinking
– difficulty making choices
– limited concentration

Intp.
– limited paralinguistic skills

Stage of group development
A group that is just beginning to enjoy a sense of cohesiveness will benefit most from this exercise.

Synopsis
The group imagines that they are seated in the basket of a hot-air balloon which is sinking. To lighten it, all but one of the passengers must jump overboard. Each person puts forward the reasons why he should be the one to be saved.

Materials and equipment
Pencils and paper.
Use a familiar room that is quiet.

Procedure

Invite everyone to sit in a circle.	To promote awareness of the group as a unit and of the individuals in it.
Pass around the paper and pencils, inviting everyone to keep one of each.	To encourage a decision on each person's part to participate actively.

---

1. This exercise is suitable for *videotaping*, particularly if the purpose of the exercise is to help patients practise more effective speaking. The replay can then be used to look at such things as: whether everyone spoke loudly enough; whether they spoke to the group as a whole or only to a segment of it; whether they were able to keep everyone's attention; whether they were able to emphasize their ideas with gestures and facial expressions.

Explain the exercise as follows:
'Imagine that we are all seated in the basket of a hot-air balloon which is sinking rapidly. The only way to prevent the balloon from crashing is to lighten it. All but one of us must jump overboard. However, since each one of us is a famous person, we are given the opportunity to put forward any reasons why we should be the one to be saved.'

'Firstly, decide which famous person you would like to be; you can be anyone either living or dead.'[2]	This part of the exercise provides each person with an opportunity to make a decision and be imaginative.
'In the next 3 minutes, write down all the arguments you can think of why you, as this famous person, should be saved.'	To assist an individual to relate his assumed identity to reality, and to encourage the use of his abilities to remember, reason and be innovative.
When the 3 minutes are up, invite one person to be the *secretary*. His job will be to write down the assumed name of each person as he speaks.	This is an opportunity to involve a quiet person in an active role.
Ask each person in turn to stand up and introduce himself to the group, using his assumed identity, and share the reasons why he considers he should be saved.[3]	This provides an opportunity to plan and practise speaking in front of a small group of people.
Encourage everyone else to listen attentively and to make notes if they wish.	To assist concentration and recall.
When everyone has spoken, a vote will be taken and the person who receives the most votes will be the winner.'	
'The *secretary* will record the votes.'	The quiet player now has an opportunity to take a leadership role in the group.
At the time of voting the therapist should remind each player that he only has one vote which he should cast for the group member whose speech contained the most persuasive reasons. Players may not vote for themselves.	This exercises decision-making.

2. The therapist should be prepared to give suggestions to those patients who do not have any ideas (see Suggestions at the end of the exercise).
3. The therapist may need to restate the reasons presented if they are very garbled. Not only will this make the person's presentation more successful, but it will also give him the feeling that he has been understood.

When all the votes have been cast, the *secretary* reads out the results.

Discussion topics
- What feelings did players experience while standing up in front of everyone and giving their speeches?
- How do players feel and react in other situations where they are expected to contribute to the conversation?
- Did your voice tone and volume make a difference to the outcome?

Suggestions for 'Save yourself'
The characters chosen can be famous politicians, comedians, singers, film stars, writers, inventors and sportsmen. They can be people who are alive today or who have died, such as:

Einstein	Michael Jordan
Shakespeare	J. F. Kennedy
Mother Theresa	Bill Clinton
John Lennon	Nelson Mandela
Napoleon	Arnold Schwarzenegger
Johann Sebastian Bach	Elvis Presley
Florence Nightingale	Bill Gates
Margaret Thatcher	Bill Cosby
King Henry VIII	

Your variations

Simultaneous conversations

Allow 30 minutes
Group size: 10 adults/6 children

This is a *theatre game* to encourage expressive self-assertion.[1]

Recommended for these problems	**Model of Human Occupation**
	Vol. – impairment of interpersonal communication as indicated by decreased eye-contact
	Perf. – difficulty speaking voluntarily due to decrease in spontaneous psychomotor behaviour
	– unassertive in social interaction
	– decreased concentration (5–15 minutes)
	Life-style Performance Model
	Sens/mo. – limited spontaneous conversation
	Cog. – short attention span
	Intp. – fear of eye-contact
	– decreased assertiveness in social situations

Stage of group development   The group members should be familiar enough with each other that they can all risk being assertive in a supportive environment.

Synopsis   Two players are assigned to be either for or against a designated topic. Then, at the same time and maintaining eye-contact, they present their point of view trying not to be distracted by their partner's argument.

Materials and equipment   None.

Procedure

Invite two players to sit facing one another...	This provides an opportunity for volunteers to come forward.
and to make eye-contact.	To assist concentration upon the other person.
The remainder of the group forms the audience.	To provide a sense of theatre.

1. The exercise is suitable for *videotaping*. The replay can be watched just for fun or to look at the specifics of being assertive. These would be such things as being able to maintain eye-contact, talk at a reasonably even pace, talk quite loudly, think quickly and creatively and not opt out of the game in any way. The nonverbal behaviour of participants can also be observed. The therapist can help the players become aware of how to reinforce what they have to say by using appropriate body positions, gestures and facial expressions.

Ask the audience to name a topic[2] (the more ridiculous it is the more amusing the exercise) … and assign[3] one of the players to be *for* it and the other to be *against*.	To encourage a sense of involvement on everyone's part and promote enjoyment.
Explain the exercise to the players as follows: 'The object of this game is to defend your assigned stand, using all the arguments you can possibly think of and to avoid responding to *any* of your opponent's monologue.[4] You do this by talking *at* one another simultaneously.'	To provide an opportunity for self-assertion and to encourage increased concentration and extemporaneous speech.
'Try to keep looking each other in the eye all the time.'	To encourage the ability to follow one train of thought without being easily distracted.
'The players will start speaking when I signal, and … 'you, the audience are the *jury*.'	
'Listen carefully to their conversations and if either of them hesitates, answers his opponent's monologue, or stops speaking altogether, call out, "hesitation".'	To encourage concentration and a sense of participation on the part of the audience.
The game then continues with a new set of players and a new topic. A discussion at the end may be appropriate.[5]	To enable all the participants to have an opportunity of experiencing the exercise. To assist self-awareness and expression of feelings evoked by the exercise.

2. In case the group is not forthcoming with any suggestions the therapist should be prepared with some alternatives (see Suggestions at the end of the exercise).
3. It may assist players who are not very self-assured if they are able to choose whether to be *for* or *against*. This is because it is often easier to defend something one believes in and has chosen to support.
4. As the players become more familiar with the exercise, encourage them to force their opponent to respond by such ruses as questions, gesticulations, laughter, etc.
5. During discussion it may be appropriate to point out that this game does not imitate normal conversation where it is always important to listen and respond to another person. However, the exercise may highlight some of the frustration that can be felt when one's conversation is ignored. It will also reinforce the importance of maintaining eye-contact when trying to keep another person interested in what one has to say and provide a chance to practise being assertive.

Discussion topics
- What did the group members think about the exercise?
- How did it make them feel?
- What does being assertive mean?
- How can a person be assertive?
- What nonverbal behaviours help a person be assertive?
- How does this exercise differ from normal interaction?

Suggestions for 'Simultaneous conversations'

Jelly beans	Olympic games
Coca Cola cans	Secondhand shoes
Doughnuts	Clearcut logging
Television programmes	Cigarette smoking
Computers	Milk
High-rise buildings	Pets
Gardening	Newspapers
Dates	Bingo
Comedians	One European currency

Your variations

Soapbox

Allow 1 hour or more
Group size: 8 adults

This is a *theatre game* to help individuals feel more comfortable when speaking in a group. It encourages decision-making and reasoning in a clear logical manner.

Recommended for these problems

Model of Human Occupation
Vol. — decreased belief in self as indicated by difficulty talking in a group situation
— diminished sense of personal effectiveness
Perf. — deficiencies in process skills as indicated by:
difficulty formulating opinions
difficulty planning

Life-style Performance Model
Cog. — difficulty making choices
Psyc. — loss of self-reliance
— fear of risking personal opinions
Intp. — limited skills in verbal group interaction

Stage of group development

The exercise should be used at a stage in group development when the participants feel fairly comfortable with one another.[1]

Synopsis

This is a modified debate in which each person makes a decision to be for or against a chosen topic and then supports it with three reasons.[2, 3]

Materials and equipment

Chairs around a table.
Prepared slips of paper (or paper and pencils).[4]
A container (hat, box, etc.).

---

1. It is contraindicated for the physically overactive patient.
2. The exercise allows each person to express opinions that he may have held when he was functioning healthily and when he relied on his own judgement. It involves short periods of concentration (while listening to the speaker) alternated with an opportunity for the expression of thoughts. It is, therefore, a useful exercise for listening, thinking and speaking.
3. The exercise can be *videotaped*. The replay can be used to look carefully at whether the participants were able to make decisions, formulate opinions and present their reasons clearly. Poor speaking habits, such as mumbling, talking very softly, talking very loudly, talking very fast or in a very hesitant way, will also become apparent. The observations made while watching the tape can form the basis for a discussion.
4. Decide whether you or the group members are to prepare the topics for discussion. This will depend on how inventive the group members can be in their choice of issues. If this task is given to the group members it may encourage them to show an active interest in community affairs (see Suggestions at the end of the exercise).

Procedure

Before beginning the exercise, list a number of controversial issues on separate slips of paper.[5] Word each one so that it can be answered by 'Yes' or 'No'. For example: 'Do you believe that there should be a minimum drinking age in pubs?'	The issues can be chosen to suit the group. Clear wording of each question will assist the speaker to think more clearly.
Invite the group to sit around a table.	This gives the group a comfortable 'boardroom' atmosphere.
Explain the exercise as follows: 'Each person will have a chance to be on the soapbox.'	To raise self-esteem, as each person will be listened to by the group.
'You will take a topic out of the hat...	This freedom of choice may discourage the suspicious person from thinking that the topic was specifically written for him.
and decide whether you are for it or against it.'	To give an opportunity for decision-making.
'Read the topic to us, tell us whether you agree or disagree with it and then back up your decision with three reasons.'[6]	This gives each person a structure around which to organize his thoughts and communicate them clearly.
In this exercise, the therapist has two jobs: (1) maintaining the freedom of speech for the speakers when necessary and (2) restating clearly what the speaker has said (if he has combined his three points into one sentence or if he has rambled). When the speaker has finished open the topic for debate.	To show the individual he has the right to speak no matter how difficult it is for him. To give him a chance to hear his thoughts clearly stated and to give him the positive feedback that he has been understood. This will encourage an interchange of ideas between two or more individuals who may otherwise find spontaneous conversation difficult.
Move on to the next person after a maximum of 10 minutes.[7, 8]	To allow time for each person to take his turn.

5. Issues which are non-threatening and of an impersonal nature are easiest for discussion. Select the types of issues in relation to the group's overall capability in handling them.
6. It may be appropriate to give each person a pencil and a slip of paper on which to note his points.
7. When there are verbose and/or hyperactive members, or if the group is large, it may be advisable to limit both the speaker's time and the open debate.
8. Do not distribute all the topics at the start, or you may find some people unable to listen to the speaker as they are concerned about how to defend their own topic best.

Discussion topics
- Why is it important to be able to make decisions?
- What are some of the problems caused by being indecisive?
- How easy or difficult was it to formulate opinions?
- What happens in a conversation when everyone is in agreement?
- What happens in a conversation when people have differing opinions?

Suggestions for 'Soapbox' topics
- Will it rain tomorrow?
- Should cars be kept out of the city centre?
- Is a welfare state essential?
- Should cigarette advertising be banned?
- Man must work to enjoy his leisure.
- Is space research important?
- Cars should be limited to one per household.
- Strikes are more effective than bargaining.

Your variations

Story-telling

Allow 1 hour
Group size: 8 adults/6 children

This is a *projective technique* that encourages creative thinking and helps individuals feel more comfortable speaking out in a group.

Recommended for these problems

Model of Human Occupation

Vol.
- decreased belief in self as indicated by difficulty with public speaking
- diminished sense of personal effectiveness as indicated by low self-confidence

Perf.
- difficulty initiating social interaction
- depression as indicated by psychomotor retardation
- deficiency in process skills as indicated by difficulty formulating ideas

Life-style Performance Model

Cog.
- loss of ability to generate ideas

Psyc.
- loss of self-reliance
- depression

Intp.
- limited skills in verbal group interaction
- limited ability to initiate conversation

Stage of group development

This exercise can be used at any stage of group cohesion.

Synopsis

In this exercise each participant makes up a simple story about a magazine picture and tells it to the group.

Materials and equipment

Magazine pictures.
Chairs around a table.

Procedure

Before beginning the exercise, collect magazines/newspaper pictures that show some action taking place, preferably where ambiguity exists so that the situation could have more than one interpretation.	This provides the visual inspiration for story-telling.
Invite the group to sit around the table and explain the purpose of the exercise.	To encourage group cohesion and eliminate the anxiety of the unknown.

Begin the exercise as follows:
'On the table are an assortment of pictures from magazines. Choose one that appeals to you.'

The choice of picture will reflect how the participant is feeling at this time.

'Look carefully at it and decide three things: What is happening now in the picture, what happened before the picture was taken, and what will happen afterwards.'[1]

This gives each person a structure to assist him organize his thoughts and communicate them clearly.

Each person is then asked in turn to tell his story.[2] Questions from the group are encouraged.

To help those who have difficulty formulating ideas.

Your variations

---

1. In reviewing this group it will become evident that what each person expressed in his story is a major issue that he is concerned with at the present time. The issue will become quickly apparent if two or more stories are chosen.
2. A variation can be added if time allows. The group chooses one picture. Then a continuous story is created with each person around the table adding on another episode until the group decides that the story is finished. It is a useful assessment tool for memory and concentration, as names, ages, and events must be remembered.

Action mime
(warm-up)

Allow up to 30 minutes
Group size: 12 adults/6 children

This *theatre game* helps a person express his ideas to others.[1]

Recommended for these problems

Model of Human Occupation
Vol.   – diminished sense of personal effectiveness
Perf.   – impairment of interpersonal communication skills as indicated by social isolation
         – decreased concentration (5 minutes or less)
         – deficiency in neurological skills as indicated by limited self-expression
         – slowing of perceptual-motor skills

Life-style Performance Model
Sens/mo. – slowed sensory-motor output
Cog.   – short attention span
Psyc.   – loss of self-reliance
         – limited self-expression
Intp.   – limited social interaction

Stage of group development

This exercise is valuable to use with any type of group, from a newly formed one to a cohesive and well integrated one.

Synopsis

Players take turns to perform an action mime, using a small article as a substitute for an imaginary one. The object of the game is to guess the identity of the imaginary article from the player's action mime.

Materials and equipment

Small articles, e.g. comb, book, box, ashtray, pencil, etc.
Use a familiar and quiet room where there will be no interruptions.

---

1. The exercise is suitable for *videotaping*. The replay will give each person a chance to see himself in action and to look at nonverbal communication skills such as effective use of hand gestures, eye-contact and the paralinguistic skills of voice tone, volume, etc. This is also an excellent exercise to videotape for those patients who are extremely anxious about the image they present.

Procedure

Invite the players to sit in a circle.	This enables each person to become more aware of the others. It also helps to unite the group.
Place a small article, e.g. a comb, in the centre of the circle.	
Explain the exercise as follows: 'In the centre of the circle I have placed a comb. In turn[2] each of us is going to pick it up and, without words, use it in such a way that our action gives it a new identity. That is, we *must not* use it as a comb, but as something else. Allow its shape, size, weight and texture to stimulate your imagination, and the rest of us will try to guess what it is from your action.'[3]	To provide an opportunity for each person to express himself and his imagination in a nonverbal manner. The game requires concentration and some spontaneity. A suitable action-mime will be immediately recognized and thus give the player a sense of achievement, whereas an inapt one will not be. The player can then be encouraged to try alternative and more realistic actions.
'Once someone in the group has guessed the identity of the imagined object correctly, place the comb back in the centre of the circle for the next person to pick up.'	The physical action of picking up or putting back the object provides each person with an opportunity to indicate nonverbally that he is either ready to take his turn or finished with it.
Continue until there are no more ideas forthcoming before substituting a different article or going on to another exercise.	Do not change the article too quickly if you wish to encourage ingenuity and imagination.

Your variations

---

2. Once everyone has had a turn, it can be useful to allow individuals to volunteer to play, especially if they need opportunities to experience decision-making and risk-taking in a supportive environment.
3. If ideas are not forthcoming, the therapist and co-therapist should be ready to act as role-models, by taking a turn first. This demonstration will also help to clarify the instructions.

Am I too close or too far away?

Allow: 1 hour
Group size: 10 adults/6 children

This exercise explores interpersonal distance in a variety of social situations.

Recommended for these problems

Model of Human Occupation
Vol.   – diminished sense of personal effectiveness
        – inability to find meaning in leisure or work
Hab.   – inability to enact meaningful roles
        – social isolation due to inappropriate habits
Perf.   – impaired nonverbal communication skills

Life-style Performance Model
Cog.   – difficulty making decisions
        – low self-confidence
Psyc.   – lowered ability to assess personal skills
Intp.   – limited nonverbal communication skills
        – limited social interaction

Stage of group development

This exercise should be done with a group of people who are familiar with one another.

Synopsis

Group members experiment with different amounts of interpersonal distance, e.g. face to face, side to side, and the application of these in different social situations such as intimate, personal and social.

Materials and equipment

12 or more 'situation cards'.
A comfortable room, with or without chairs.

Procedure

Ask everyone to stand in a circle.	This places everyone in a position of physical readiness.
Explain the exercise as follows: 'We are going to do an exercise that explores the distances we put between ourselves and others in a variety of different social situations.'	A simple explanation reduces anxiety.
'Is there one person who would like to volunteer to stand in the centre of the circle?'	An opportunity for someone to assume a leadership role and engage in some risk taking.

'We will take turns to walk slowly towards the centre person until we get "too close for comfort".'	To become aware of physical distance between people.
'When you reach that point, stop and say. "This is too close for me".'	To make a personal decision and share it.
'Ask the centre person if it is too close for her as well.'	To ascertain if both individuals feel the same or different.
'Then take one or more small steps back until you feel you are at a comfortable distance and say, "This feels right for me".'	To identify your dimensions of your comfort zone.
'Ask the centre person if it feels good for her and if it does stop there and measure how far apart you are, using your arms.'	This assists a person to identify the distance using her body – arms length is a common comfortable distance between people in face to face situations.
'Does everyone understand what we are going to do?'	To provide an opportunity for anyone who did not understand to ask for clarification.
Invite someone to be the first volunteer. Guide each person through the procedure, asking the centre person to face each person as they begin their walk and to make eye-contact.	
When the whole group is standing around the centre person, say: 'Let's look around and see how the distance that feels comfortable varies from person to person.'	
'Now turn sideways to the centre person and move closer/farther away until you reach your comfortable distance.'	The physical action keeps everyone involved in the exercise.
'Consider if this is the same distance as before or a different one?'	To compare face to face distance with side by side.
Once this part of the exercise has been done, ask everyone to sit down in a circle and introduce a discussion on 'interpersonal distance'.	
Following this, invite each person to take a 'situation card' and study the type of social interaction occurring.	To take the information and use it in becoming more aware of different types of social situations.

Each person then tells the group what the card says, identifies the type of social interaction and physically arranges two or more people at the distance that feels right for the situation.

This helps group members become aware that interpersonal distance changes according to the type of social interaction.

Encourage group participants to comment on the comfort levels and situational appropriateness of the distances they are placed in.[1]

This encourages social interaction.

Discussion topics	– Our individual personal space bubble, how big/small is it, does it change and if so under what circumstances?
	– What distances are appropriate in social situations?
	– When we stand too close to someone how do they feel?
	– When we make mistakes in interpersonal distance as related to the type of social interaction we are engaging in, what are the possible consequences?
	– Besides distance, what other nonverbal behaviours change with the type of interaction, e.g. voice loudness, eye-contact, gestures.
Suggestions for situation cards	Identify the type of social interaction occurring and arrange two group members the appropriate distance for this type of conversation:

Calling a friend on the telephone to arrange to meet for coffee
Playing a card game with a partner
An acquaintance is telling you about one of her children bedwetting
You have lost your job and want to tell your wife
Your son is feeling downhearted about a poor test result
Your daughter asks to talk to you about boyfriend problems
You give your daughter a hug
Saying goodbye to a work mate
Saying goodbye to your husband
You feel depressed and are telling a close friend
An acquaintance borrowed a book. You ask for it back
Two friends in the playground sharing a secret
A group of friends having a chat
A group of people standing talking at a convention
A group of people at a party

Your variations

Edward Hall,[1] in his book *The Hidden Dimension*, suggests the following guidelines can be considered:
1. *Intimate zone.* Up to 18 inches (almost touching). Used with close friends and family members for intimate conversation. Voice quiet to very quiet, topics personal.
   Personal zone. Between 18 inches and 4 feet. Used for social conversation with friends and family. Voice not too loud, topics varied, but not too personal.
   Social zone. Between 4 and 12 feet. Used with anyone. Appropriate to talk loudly so others can hear. Topics are superficial.

REFERENCES

1. Hall, Edward T. (1966) *The Hidden Dimension.* New York: Doubleday.

Allow: 30–60 minutes
Group size: 10 adults/6 children

Charades
(Adapted from Norwicki and Duke.[1])

This *theatre game* is used to practise the nonverbal communication skills of facial expression, gestures and body posture.

Recommended for these problems

Model of Human Occupation

Vol.	– diminished sense of personal effectiveness
	– loss of internal locus of control
Hab.	– inability to enact meaningful roles
	– social isolation due to dysfunctional habits
Perf.	– impaired nonverbal communication skills

Life-style Performance Model

Cog.	– short attention span
Psyc.	– loss of self-esteem
Intp.	– limited social interaction
	– limited nonverbal communication skills

Stage of group development

This exercise is suitable to use with a group who have not met together very many times. It encourages group cohesion.

Synopsis

The group divides into two teams, who take turns to mime a selected feeling using a particular type of body language for the other team to identify.

Materials and equipment

3 sets of cards:
    20 Feeling cards.
    10 Method cards.
    10 Send/Receive cards.
(See Suggestions at the end of the exercise)
A comfortable room with chairs.

Procedure

Before this exercise make up the 3 sets of cards.

Divide the group into two teams.[1]	
Invite the teams to sit at opposite ends of the room and select a leader.	This provides an opportunity for someone to assume a responsible role.
The therapist or a group member shuffles each of the 3 sets of cards and places them face down in front of the teams.	This provides an opportunity to involve a group member in a physical way.

Explain the exercise as follows:	
'We are going to do an exercise that is a variation of the game Charades.'	Relating the exercise to a game that is familiar will help to relieve any anxiety group members may have.

'We have three piles of cards here.	
The leader of each team picks a card from the send/receive pile.	
If the card says "send" then she picks up a "method" card and a "feeling" card and quietly shares the words with the team.'	

The whole team, after discussing their mime, act out the feeling in the indicated way, e.g. feeling – optimistic, method – posture and walk, for the other team to guess.'	Working in a group will encourage social interaction between the team members and the synchronizing of the nonverbal skill to be enacted.

'If the leader of your team picks up a "receive" card then the other team must pick up a "feeling" and "method" card and act it out.	The surprise element will encourage adaptability and help to maintain interest.
The other team will call out their answers.'	

'Hand gestures can be used by the miming team leader or all her group members to indicate if the guesses are getting close.'	To encourage the use of gestures for the purpose of interactive communication.

'Once your team guesses the feeling correctly, then you receive a point.'	The competitive element will assist in developing team spirit.

'Does anyone have any questions?'	To provide an opportunity for anyone who has not understood the instructions to ask for them to be repeated.

'The teams will alternate turns for picking from the send/receive pile.'	
If you wish, the position of leader can move to other members of the team.	To provide an opportunity for all group members to try out the leadership role.

---

1. The exercise can be adapted for individuals to do the mimes rather than the whole team if the group members trust one another enough to begin risk taking.

Discussion
  – How important is it to be able to express our feelings nonverbally?
  – Which of the 'methods' did you find easiest or most difficult?
  – Can a person learn to express himself more effectively using nonverbal language skills? If so, how?
  – How did you feel as the team leader?

Suggestions for cards
  Feeling cards. Bored, angry, sad, happy, excited, apprehensive, afraid, proud, shy, enthusiastic, calm, brave, optimistic, worried, guilty, scared, sulky, lonely, playful, exhausted, hurt, elated, fascinated, sympathetic, thoughtful.
  Method cards. Each one with one or two words describing body language, e.g. facial expression, touch, hand gesture, body posture, walk, rhythm, eye-contact.
  Send/Receive cards. Print 5 of each.

Your variations

REFERENCES

1. Norwicki, S., Duke, M. (1992) *Helping the Child who Doesn't Fit In.* Atlanta: Peachtree Publishers.

Cooperation

Allow: 30 minutes
Group size: 10 adults/6 children

(Adapted from Stalker.[1])

This is a problem-solving exercise making use of nonverbal communication skills.

Recommended for these problems

Model of Human Occupation

Vol.   – impairment of interpersonal communication skills as indicated by social anxiety

Perf. – difficulty problem solving
     – deficient nonverbal skills in the following domains:
        facial expression and eye-contact
        posture and gestures
        interpersonal distance and touch

Life-style Performance Model

Cog. – difficulty problem solving

Intp. – limited interpersonal skills
     – limited nonverbal skills in the following areas:
        facial expression and eye-contact
        posture and gestures
        interpersonal distance and touch

Stage of group development

This is a good exercise to use with a group of people who have worked together for a few sessions and who are beginning to trust one another.

Synopsis

Two people stand at opposite ends of a line on the floor. They must find a way to change places, without knocking each other off the line.

Materials and equipment

Roll of wide masking tape or piece of chalk.
Large comfortable room.

Procedure

Tape or draw a 2 metre line on the floor approximately 10 cm wide.

Explain the exercise as follows:
'The taped line represents a very narrow bridge over a deep and muddy river full of ...' (use examples such as snakes, alligators, slugs, etc., or whatever is suitable for the age range of the group members).

The taped line is a symbol to help the participants visualize the situation.

Children, particularly those who are more reticent, can be asked to suggest what scary creatures are in the water, as a way of encouraging them to participate in the exercise.

'We are going to work in pairs and start by standing at opposite ends of the "bridge". We both want to cross over to the other side at the same time but we cannot speak. The problem we have to solve is how to pass one another on the bridge without falling into the river and without using words to communicate? If you lose your balance and fall into the river we will all come to your rescue.'	To provide an opportunity for the two individuals to use eye-contact, facial expression and gestures to communicate.
'Does everyone understand what we are going to do?' Number off the group members into pairs – 1, 2, 3, 4, 1, 2, 3, 4, etc. – and then ask…	To allow for clarification of the instructions and purpose.
'Who would like to go first?'	This provides an opportunity for two people to demonstrate initiative.
Observe each pair and their problem-solving strategies and use of nonverbal language skills, such as facial expression, hand gestures, etc.	Make notes if need be as a memory jog for the discussion later.
Invite the group members to cheer on the efforts of each pair to solve the problem. If a pair fall off the bridge, encourage everyone to get involved in the rescue. This can be particularly fun with children and is a way of involving everyone in a cooperative exercise.	
When every pair have had a turn, sit down in a circle and have a discussion.	To reunite the group.

Discussion topics
- Discuss the various different strategies that each couple used and which worked best.
- Explore cooperative methods versus others
- Which were the best, most creative, easiest to execute solutions and why?
- What happens to communication when you cannot speak?
- Is it easier or more difficult to problem solve when you cannot speak? Elaborate.

- Are there any more solutions to this particular problem that were not tried?
- How does a person's ability to solve problems affect day to day life?
- Can most problems be solved in several different ways? How does one choose which would be the most effective solution?
- Would you like to try this exercise again, this time using words to assist in the problem solving process?

Your variations

REFERENCES

1. Stalker, A. (1991) *Bridges to Competence, Activities for Theme-based Social Skills Groups.* Available from the Occupational Therapy Department, British Columbia's Children's Hospital, 4480 Oak St., Vancouver, B.C., V6H 3V4, Canada.

Expressions

Allow 1–1½ hours
Group size: 8 adults/6 children

This is an exercise which illustrates the part facial expression plays in communication between people.[1]

Recommended for these problems

Model of Human Occupation
Vol. – limited self-concept
– blunted affect
– decreased belief in self as indicated by difficulty talking in a group situation
– loss of self-esteem
Perf. – decreased concentration (5 minutes or less)[2]

Life-style Performance Model
Cog. – short attention span
Psyc. – lowered ability to assess personal skills
– flat affect
– loss of self-esteem
Intp. – limited skills in verbal group interaction

Stage of group development

This is an excellent exercise for a group of withdrawn, depressed people. The group members need not know one another very well but some familiarity may be helpful if they are to work together easily.

Synopsis

The group members make a collage of faces which show a variety of expressions. They identify the different feelings portrayed and then each person mimes one of the feelings for the group to guess.

Materials and equipment

A wide variety of magazines.
Scissors.
Glue.
A large sheet of paper (e.g. 60 cm × 90 cm) (on a separate table).
Felt pens.
Small slips of paper and a container.
Room which is large enough to provide adequate working space.

---

1. The second and third parts of this exercise are suitable for *videotaping*. When the replay is watched players will be able to see their own attempts at using their faces to express feelings. The replay will also bring into focus the fact that besides facial expression, feelings can be effectively communicated using body posture, body movements and gestures.
2. The fact that the exercise is composed of three distinct parts means that it tends to re-focus the attention of patients who have difficulty maintaining contact with reality for long periods of time.

Procedure

Invite the group members to gather around the table.	To encourage a sense of group cohesiveness.
Give the following instructions: 'From the magazines provided, select and cut out a number of faces of people.'	To promote active individual participation and exercise the capacities of choice and motor coordination.
(Sometimes it is useful to limit the number of faces to be selected by each person, e.g. 2 or 5.)	To give the participants limits within which to work and help to reduce any anxiety arising through the tendency to be overinclusive. If the group is large and the attention span of the members short, this will also ensure that the collage contains a reasonable amount of resource material and yet represents each person.
'Try to choose a variety of expressions.'	To encourage discrimination through paying attention to detail as well as to assist recall of the wide range of emotions.
'When you have made your selection, paste these faces on the paper to form a collage.'[3]	To encourage goal-directed behaviour and cooperative interaction with the other participants.
When this part of the exercise has been completed explain the next part: 'We now need two volunteers, a leader and a secretary.'	To provide an opportunity for transferring leadership from the therapist to the group members.
'The leader will select one of the faces on the collage and point to it. He will invite the rest of us to decide what feeling or feelings we consider the face is expressing.'	This requires decisions by both the leader and participants, together with mutual cooperation. It provides a check for the accuracy of individual perceptions.
'When the majority of us agree, the secretary will record this feeling on a slip of paper, which he will fold and place in a container.'	'To help the leader exercise his diplomacy and ability to recognize a final or majority decision.

---

3. You can choose one or two people to paste the faces on to the paper. It is best if this job is given either to a person who feels cutting out pictures is beneath him or to a person who is restless. It provides an opportunity for leadership and making decisions.

Inviting the group to gather around the collage, proceed with the exercise until all or most of the faces have been discussed.	To give an opportunity to be aware of a wide range of feelings.
Then remove the collage and ask the group to sit in a circle.	This physical activity tends to promote renewed interest.
In turn, invite each person to pick one of the slips of paper out of the container and mime the feeling written on it, for the group to guess.	To provide an opportunity for each person to experiment with the use of a larger range of facial expressions for which he receives recognition and feedback.
At the end, ask the group members if they have any comments on the exercise.	To encourage the participants to discuss the importance of observing and understanding facial expression as an aid to successful communication.

Discussion topics
- The ease or difficulty with which the participants were able to mime emotions.
- How any particular facial expression may affect others and thus our relationships.
- In what other ways do we express feelings nonverbally?

Your variations   A suggested variation is to ask group members (individually, in pairs, or in groups) to find pictures of faces to illustrate some or all of the following feelings: boredom, trust, repulsion, relief, loneliness, hate, joy, anger, fear, contentment, strength, unfulfilment, support, confusion, shyness, inferiority, involvement, frustration, superiority, suspicion, attraction, hurt, love, sadness, affection, hope, weakness, satisfaction, rejection, or curiosity. This would be valuable for patients who need more structure and/or whose descriptive abilities are severely impaired. Discussion could be based on comparing and contrasting the pictures each group found to illustrate similar feelings or on the appropriateness of the pictures selected.

Allow: 10–20 minutes
Group size: 12 adults/6 children

Join me (warm-up)

(Adapted from Stalker.[1])

This is a nonverbal activity that explores the use of facial expression, eye-contact, gestures and posture in social situations. This exercise would be an excellent one to *videotape*.

Recommended for these problems

Model of Human Occupation

Vol.
- limited self-concept
- loss of internal locus of control
- difficulty differentiating and expressing feelings

Perf.
- impairment of interpersonal communication skills as indicated by social isolation

Life-style Performance Model

Psyc.
- lowered ability to assess personal skills
- difficulty differentiating and expressing feelings

Intp.
- limited social interaction
- limited receptive and expressive nonverbal skills

Stage of group development

This exercise is suitable to use with a new group as a warm-up. If it is used to generate an in-depth discussion regarding nonverbal language skills and their use, then the group members should know and trust one another.

Synopsis

A person stands at one end of the room and tries to persuade everyone to join him by using nonverbal language only.

Materials and equipment

None.
Use a comfortable, carpeted room.

Procedure

Ask everyone to sit down on the floor in a group and then explain the exercise as follows:	This physically unites the group to begin the session.
'Today we are going to begin with a warm-up that explores the way we use nonverbal language skills. Do you know what I mean by nonverbal language skills?'	The explanation gives the exercise a focus and relieves anxiety. This allows for individuals to ask for clarification.
Be ready to discuss examples of nonverbal communication such as gestures and posture, facial expression and eye-contact.	To help individuals become aware of the variety of nonverbal communications they can use.

'One of us will volunteer to stand at the other
end of the room and, without using words, try to
persuade all of us to join him.'[1]

'Who would like to be first?'

This provides an opportunity for a person to
volunteer in a leadership role.

The therapist should volunteer if participants are
reluctant.
Instruct the group members to join when they
feel welcome.
Coaching or modelling may be necessary to assist
the participants think about the ways in which
they can use their bodies to communicate
effectively.

Once one member has had a turn, encourage
everyone else to take turns and then either move
into another exercise or discuss how the exercise
went.

Discussion topics
- Is nonverbal language an important part of communication?
- What happens if your nonverbal language skills are poor?
- Which types of nonverbal skills were the most successful in this group? Why?
- Do we communicate when we sit quietly in a group of people and say nothing? If so, how and what do we communicate?
- What happens to communication when the words and the non-verbal message are different? Can you think of examples?
- How did it feel to be alone and trying to persuade everyone to join you?
- How did it feel to be the only one not to join the group? What were your reasons for not joining?

Your variations

REFERENCES

1. Stalker, A. (1991) *Bridges to Competence, Activities for Theme-based Social Skills Groups.* Available from the Occupational Therapy Department, British Columbia's Children's Hospital, 4480 Oak St., Vancouver, B.C., V6H 3V4, Canada.

Allow 15–30 minutes
Group size: 8 adults/6 children

Magic box

This is a *theatre game* that requires nonverbal communication. It may assist an individual to improve his concentration and memory.[1]

Recommended for these problems

Model of Human Occupation

Vol.	– inhibited self-expression due to decreased expectations of success
	– inability to make decisions
Perf.	– decreased concentration as indicated by forgetfulness
	– slowing of perceptual-motor skills

Life-style Performance Model

Sens/mo.	– difficulty processing sensory information
Cog.	– difficulty making choices
	– short attention span
	– diminished retention and recall
	– inhibited self-expression

Stage of group development

This exercise is best used with a small group of people; they need not be familiar with one another.

Synopsis

Each player, in turn, mimes an object and places it in an imaginary box. He then mimes all the other imaginary objects the box contains that were placed there by preceding players.

Materials and equipment

None.
Use a familiar room that is carpeted.

Procedure

Invite the group members to sit on the floor in a circle of less than 10 people.[2]	To form a small unit of people who will feel at ease working together.
Designate a leader in each group, or, if the exercise is familiar, invite volunteers to take the position of leader in the group.	

1. This exercise is suitable for *videotaping*. The replay will be fun to watch and will allow each person to see his ability to be creative and uninhibited.
2. The amount of information that each person has to memorize is directly proportionate to the number of people; if the attention span of the participants is short it is advisable that the group be divided into smaller units.

Explain the exercise as follows:

'The leader will mime an imaginary box (its shape, size, weight, and texture, etc.) which he will produce and place on the floor in front of him.'	To provide an opportunity for creative self-expression.
'He will open it and take out an imaginary object which he will use in such a way that its identity is obvious to the rest of us.'	To encourage contact with reality by recalling the use of familiar objects and to practise nonverbal communication.
'Then he will place the object in the box, close the lid, and pass it on to the next person.'[3]	To enable each person in the group to participate.
'This player will open the box, remove the imagined object and use it in the same or a different manner...'	This part of the exercise requires memory, self-expression and concentration.
'then, placing it back in the box, he will take out his own mime object which he will use and place in the box too.'	To give an opportunity to practise making choices.
'Closing the lid he will pass the box on to the next player.'[4]	To encourage interaction between the two people.
The box continues around the circle with each person using all of the previously invented objects and then adding one of his own.	As the game progresses, there is an increasing amount of concentration, memory and initiative required on the part of each successive person.
When the box finally returns to the leader, he removes all the objects one by one, uses them and then throws them away.	To conclude the game symbolically.

Discussion topics
– The ease/difficulty of using nonverbal language skills to communicate.
– What specific skills did you need to use – facial expression, posture, hand gestures, eye-contact, etc.
– When do you use nonverbal communication during your daily life?
– Do you find it easy to interpret other people's facial expressions, body posture, etc. so that you know what they are feeling?

Your variations

---

3. If the players are at all confused, specify the direction in which they pass the box (e.g. 'Pass the box to the person on your right.')
4. The therapist (leader) may need to remind the participants to remember the size, shape and weight of the box, as well as the contents.

Allow 5–15 minutes
Group size: 10 adults/6 children

Mirrors

This is an exercise to help a person improve his ability to communicate and interact with another person.[1]

Recommended for these problems

Model of Human Occupation

Vol.   – impairment of interpersonal communication as indicated by:

decreased eye-contact

social isolation

– distorted body image

– inhibited self-expression due to decreased expectations of success

Perf.   – decreased concentration (5–15 minutes)

– limited nonverbal communcation skills

Life-style Performance Model

Sens/mo. – distorted body image

Cog.   – short attention span

Psyc.   – inhibited self-expression

Intp.   – fear of eye contact

– limited social interaction

Stage of group development

This is an appropriate exercise to use when there is little interaction between group members.

Synopsis

Two people stand facing one another and mirror each other's movements. They take turns being leader or follower. Finally they continue moving and reflecting one another with neither one consciously leading.

Materials and equipment

None required.[2]

Use a familiar room that is quiet.

---

1. The exercise is suitable for *videotaping*. The replay will enable the participants to see how they reacted during the exercise. They will be able to view their emotional and physical responses in the two different roles.
2. However, this exercise could be done using music as a means of suggesting patterns of movement to the participants. For musical suggestions refer to the exercise *Painting to music*, p. 167.

Procedure

Invite the group members to divide into pairs, choosing a partner with whom they feel at ease, and with whom they would like to work.	This is to encourage each person to become aware of the other group members and to contact one of them in particular.
Explain the exercise as follows: 'Stand about 1 metre away from your partner, look him in the eye, then look away. Do this several times until you are more comfortable.'	For those people who find making and maintaining eye-contact very difficult it is important that they have a chance to practise. If everyone does the exercise simultaneously it will help those who are at all self-conscious.
'When you both feel comfortable, decide between you who will be the leader and who will be the follower.'	This requires cooperation and decision-making between the two people.
'Then, looking each other in the eye as continuously as possible...'	Maintaining eye-contact requires considerable concentration.
'I would like the leader to start moving his body or a part of it *very, very slowly.*' (Stress the last part.)	This provides an opportunity for a person to lead and initiate actions, in a controlled and deliberate way.
'At the same time as you do this your partner will try to mirror your action exactly.'	To enable a person to observe his own body movements as reflected by his partner. This requires concentration and will exercise his ability to perceive and mime body movements.
Allow each pair to practise, giving assistance or demonstration where it is necessary.	To encourage everyone to become involved in the doing of the exercise and to assist them in carrying out the instructions correctly.
Then invite the pairs to switch roles, so that the leader becomes the follower and vice versa.	This enables everyone to experience both roles, and may encourage versatility.
When each pair has switched roles several times, continue by giving the following instructions: 'Now I would like you to move in free form, that is, with neither one of you consciously leading or following and yet each of you continuing to mirror the movements of the other.'	This encourages sensitivity to another person and the experience of working simultaneously with him; it also requires greater concentration.
When the exercise is over, ask the group members to sit in a circle.	
Invite them to discuss any feelings or reactions they may have experienced.	To encourage the sharing of feelings evoked by this experience of nonverbal interaction.

Discussion topics
- How did it feel to make eye-contact with another person?
- Was it easy or difficult to maintain eye-contact?
- For what percentage of a conversation would you make eye-contact?
- Discuss the importance of looking at people in order to communicate more effectively.
- Discuss people's rhythms. Are they all the same? How can you discern a person's rhythm?
- Should we try and match other people's rhythms and what are the social consequences of doing or not doing this?

Your variations

Allow 15–30 minutes
Group size: 12 adults/6 children

Movement and sound circle (warm-up)

This is a *theatre game* requiring self-expression, communication, and interaction.[1]

Recommended for these problems

Model of Human Occupation

Vol.   – inhibited self expression due to decreased expectations of success
          – lack of awareness of body movements
Perf.   – slowing of perceptual-motor skills
          – limited nonverbal communication skills

Life-style Performance Model

Sens/mo. – slowed sensory motor output
          – decreased body awareness
          – decreased nonverbal communication skills
Psyc.   – inhibited self-expression

Stage of group development

This is an appropriate exercise for a group in which the members find communication difficult.

Synopsis

One player stands in the centre of a circle and initiates a repetitive movement with an associated sound. He then teaches his movement/sound to another player. The two people then exchange positions and the new player develops the movement/sound into a different movement/sound and passes it on.

Materials and equipment

None.
Use a familiar room that is quiet.

Procedure

Invite the group members to stand in a circle.	This enables each person to see and, therefore, be more aware of everyone else.
Explain the exercise as follows: 'One person stands in the centre of the circle and...'[2, 3]	To provide a focus for the attention of the group members.

1. The exercise is suitable for *videotaping*. The replay can be watched just for fun and will allow participants to see themselves creating uninhibited body movement and associated sounds.

'initiates a repetitive movement, and in conjunction with it – a fitting sound.'[4, 5, 6]	To provide an opportunity for self-expression in the form of repetitive physical activity and simple verbalization.
'When the movement and sound have evolved to his satisfaction...'[7]	
'he moves to stand in front of one of the players in the surrounding circle.'	To encourage awareness of others and provide an opportunity to make a choice from a selection of alternatives.
'He teaches his movement/sound to this person.'[8]	To encourage nonverbal communication.
'The player being taught tries to imitate both the action and the sound as closely as he can.'[9]	To encourage interaction while concentrating upon another person. To assist body awareness, since both the individuals are receiving visual feedback on how their actions appear.
'When the teacher is satisfied that his movement/ sound have been learned accurately, the two players change positions.	

2. If the game is being played for the first time, the therapist is advised to take this position in order to demonstrate the instructions he gives. If, however, the players are familiar with the exercise, ask if there is a volunteer who would like to be in the centre of the circle. This provides an opportunity for someone to demonstrate initiative.

3. If the players are hesitant to be the only person in the centre, because it means they are the focus of everyone's attention, it may be advisable to begin with two or even three people there. Each one of them teaches his own 'movement and sound' simultaneously.

4. With some groups (e.g. those who find it difficult to cope with more than one idea at a time), simplify the exercise. Begin with the movements and include the sounds as the group members become relaxed.

5. Encourage the players to keep the actions large and the sounds simple and loud, since they are easier to imitate and tend to be more stimulating, e.g. marching to the sound 'boom', 'boom', 'boom'.

6. As the players become more proficient, they may be encouraged to introduce words and phrases instead of simple sounds. A question and answer situation may develop or even a continuing story.

7. Ideally the movement and sound should evolve naturally to suit the person in the centre of the circle. Therefore, the therapist must discourage him from stopping to think, fumble or wonder 'What shall I do?'

8. If the whole group imitates the action and sound as it is being taught this will encourage both an enthusiastic and energetic response. It may also help to keep the energy level up during the evolution of new action and sounds and tend to give the central player encouragement and support.

9. Encourage the action and sound to be repeated over and over again until the player can imitate them to the best of his ability.

'The new player takes his learned movement/ sound into the centre of the circle where he allows them to develop (by exaggerating or distorting the sound and movement) into a different movement/sound of his own making.'

He then teaches his own movement/sound to another player and so the exercise progresses.	To enable everyone to take part in the exercise. The random choice of who goes into the centre of the circle tends to increase the spontaneity and is less anxiety-provoking than waiting to go in a particular order.
After the exercise is over you may like to invite the group members to discuss briefly their reactions to the exercise. If this exercise is used as a warm-up, discussion is more appropriate at the end of the entire session.	To encourage expression of feelings evoked by the exercise.

Discussion topics — Discussion can be introduced following this exercise on the subject of nonverbal communication. The exercise touches on all of the following: personal rhythm, interpersonal distance, use of posture and gestures, facial expression and eye-contact as well as combining these with the paralinguistic skills of voice tone, volume, pitch and synchronicity. Any one of these could be discussed in greater detail.

Your variations

Mystery objects

Allow 10–30 minutes
Group size: 10 adults/6 children

This is a *theatre game* that stimulates tactile perception.

Recommended for these problems

Model of Human Occupation
Vol.   – decreased belief in self as indicated by:
                 loss of self-esteem
                 difficulty talking in a group situation
Perf.   – difficulty interpreting sensory cues
Life-style Performance Model
Sens/mo. – decreased visual/tactile discrimination
Psyc.   – loss of self-esteem
             – difficulty sustaining contact with external stimuli
Intp.   – limited interpersonal skills

Stage of group development

This exercise is useful for a group whose members have difficulty talking to one another.

Synopsis

A player is given a small article to hold behind his back and by using his sense of touch, tries to answer questions about the article and guess its identity.

Materials and equipment

Container.
20 small articles.

Procedure

Beforehand, invite all the players to bring a number of small articles.	To encourage a sense of responsibility and involvement in the group's activities.
Prior to beginning the game, pass the container around for each person to place his contributions in, without revealing them to the others.	
Then invite the players to sit down in a circle and ask if there is a volunteer willing to stand up in front of everybody.	To provide an opportunity for a group member to take a risk in a warm supportive environment.

Explain the exercise as follows:
'The volunteer stands with his back to the group and his hands behind him.'

'The leader takes an object out of the bag and places it in the hands of the volunteer.' Once the therapist has demonstrated how the game is played, the position of *leader* can be taken by a group member.

'He then asks the volunteer six or seven questions about the article (e.g. "What shape is it?" "What size is it?" "How does it feel?" and amusing questions, such as "What colour do you think it is?" and finally "Do you know what the article is?")'	To provide the volunteer with an opportunity to arrive at a decision using tactile discrimination and deduction. If seated, group members are encouraged also to think of questions to ask as this will help them to feel more involved.
'The volunteer attempts to answer these to the best of his ability, without looking.' (As the group can see the article some of the questions and answers can be very amusing).	To improve tactile perception and verbal interaction related to an everyday object.
After a given number of questions (e.g. 10), the volunteer is invited to look at the object before placing it back in the bag. He then returns to his place in the circle.	So that he can compare his visual perception with what he sensed by touch.
Encourage the audience to applaud and then invite another volunteer to come forward.[1]	To increase self-esteem by providing a rewarding and supportive conclusion to his turn.

Your variations

---

1. This exercise can be adapted for patients who are very withdrawn and isolated. If simple, everyday objects are used, the chances of success in identification are considerably increased.

People machine

This *theatre game* encourages physical closeness in an enjoyable way. It can be used as a *warm-up* or a longer activity.

Recommended for these problems	**Model of Human Occupation**
	Vol. – impairment of interpersonal communication as indicated by:
	        difficulty trusting people
	        social isolation
	Perf. – slowing of perceptual-motor skills
	        – impairment of interpersonal communication skills as indicated by fear of touching people
	Life-style Performance Model
	Sens/mo. – slowed sensory-motor output
	Intp. – limited capacity for trust
	        – limited social interaction
	        – fear of physical contact

Stage of group development	This is a good exercise to use with a group who are getting to know one another.[1]
Synopsis	The group members join together to make a piece of moving machinery with as many moving gears and levers as they can think of.
Materials and equipment	None. A comfortable, carpeted room would be appropriate.

Procedure

Invite everyone to stand in a circle.	To bring the group together.
Explain the exercise as follows: 'We are going to make a piece of moving machinery.'	To give an overall picture of the activity.
'One of us will begin by standing in the centre of the circle.'	To provide an opportunity for someone to assume leadership.

---

1. This exercise is not recommended to be used with people with schizophrenia who are fearful of close encounters.

'This person will think of a movement and sound
that represents a small part of a large machine.'

'When he is ready he will make this movement and sound repetitively.'	This allows the person to express ideas in a physical manner.
'Watch him closely to get a clear idea of what he is doing.'	To re-focus the attention of group members.
'Then think of a movement and sound of your own.'	Some people may need encouragement at this time.
'When you are ready, move into the centre of the circle, and...'	To encourage personal decision-making
'attach yourself in some way to another person.'	It is important that the participants link up with one another physically.
'Then begin making your own movement and sound.'	This provides an opportunity to interact with the group nonverbally.
'Try to keep in mind that we are making a large piece of machinery.'	Continuous re-focusing of the purpose of the exercise helps those who have a short attention span.

Discussion topics
- Did the machine have a purpose, beginning or end?
- Did it produce anything and, if so, what?
- Is it important that we associate with other people and work together?
- Do we need to link up with people in our lives and, if so, in what situations is it appropriate?
- How does it feel to be physically close to other people?
- Is it easy or difficult to be close to others?

Your variations

Allow 5–30 minutes
Group size: 10 adults/6 children

Sort yourself out
(warm-up)
(Adapted from Stalker.[1])

This is an exercise to develop awareness of oneself and others.

Recommended for these problems

Model of Human Occupation
Vol.   – limited self-concept and inability to make decisions
         – loss of internal locus of control as indicated by:
             lack of insight
             difficulty differentiating feelings
Hab.   – role imbalance
Perf.   – unassertive in social interaction
Life-style Performance Model
Cog.   – difficulty making choices
Psyc.   – lowered ability to assess personal skills
         – difficulty understanding and expressing feelings
Intp.   – decreased assertiveness in social situations

Stage of group development

This exercise is appropriate for a group that achieved some sense of group identity. It is a valuable exercise to use as a warm-up or to introduce if group energy is low.

Synopsis

The group subdivides by identifying similarities and differences of both physical characteristics, interests and personality traits. The process is repeated a number of times moving from concrete to more abstract concepts.

Materials and equipment

Masking tape.
A comfortable room, with enough space for group members to move around freely.

Procedure

Tape a 3 metre line on the floor. Invite everyone in the group to stand up.	The physical movement encourages an attitude of readiness for the exercise.

The therapist stands at one end of the line. Explain the exercise as follows: 'I am going to call out two descriptive words. Think about which one describes you best.'[1]	To encourage self-awareness.
'For example, all those of you wearing light colours stand on my right forming one group and those of you who are wearing dark colours, stand on my left forming a second group.'	Giving a concrete example will relieve anxiety.
Enquire if everyone understands.	This allows anyone who was not listening to ask for instructions to be repeated.
'Go ahead and form your groups and then take a few seconds to notice who is wearing the same colour as you. 'Now look at the variations of colour within your group.'	To encourage everyone to look for small similarities and differences even within their own group.
'Next we'll use a different criterion – those of you who are 5 feet 6 inches tall or more form a group on my right and those of you who are 5 feet 5 inches tall or less form a group on my left.	This demonstrates that group composition can change depending upon the criteria.
'Sit down for a minute in your group.'	To physically unite the group.
'Let's think about some issues around the subject of height. Do you all like being the height you are? Does being tall or short have an impact on your life? If so, how? The discussion can be widened at this point to include both groups.	Generating discussion assists members to share thoughts, feelings, etc. on a common characteristic.
'Now let's use yet another criterion. Those of you who like watching sports on T.V., form a group on my right and those of you who do not, form a group on my left.' Continue in this manner, using categories that are appropriate for the age, interests, etc. of the participants.	

1. Start with physical characteristics such as height, colour or type of hair, etc. Proceed to superficial personal issues such as likes and dislikes, food preferences, hobbies, interests, etc. and finally, if appropriate, to personality traits, beliefs and life situations such as happy/sad, quiet/noisy, quick/slow, never gets angry/often does, worries a lot/doesn't worry much, optimistic/pessimistic, marital or employment status, being a child of divorced parents, amount of friends/interests outside the institution, etc.

Encourage discussion around each issue as is appropriate by exploring these descriptive categories in greater depth.

By becoming more aware of similarities and differences, group members are able to share feelings and become more supportive of one another.

Discussion topics
– What are the positive and negative aspects of descriptive words and categories?
– Is it comforting to be similar to others? Why?
– How important are looks, age, interests, etc., when making friends?
– Should we draw conclusions about people from their physical characteristics?

Your variations

REFERENCES

1. Stalker, A. (1991) *Bridges to Competence, Activities for Theme-based Social Skills Groups.* Available from the Occupational Therapy Department, British Columbia's Children's Hospital, 4480 Oak St., Vancouver, B.C., V6H 3V4, Canada.

<table>
<tr><td>Allow 1 hour
Group size: 8 adults/6 children</td><td></td></tr>
</table>

Theme collage

This is an exercise to promote group cohesion through the nonverbal and verbal interaction which occurs when a group of people work together.

Recommended for these problems	**Model of Human Occupation**
	Vol. – impairment of interpersonal communication skills as indicated by: social anxiety inability to make decisions
	Hab. – feelings of incompetence
	Perf. – decreased social involvement – limited task-oriented skills – difficulty planning

Life-style Performance Model

Cog. – difficulty making choices
Psyc. – feelings of anxiety
Intp. – limited interpersonal skills
– withdrawal from reciprocal interpersonal relationships

Stage of group development This is a valuable exercise to use with a group that lacks cohesion and contains a number of very isolated members.

Synopsis The group choose a theme together and then compose a collage which represents each person's perception of that theme.

Materials and equipment Magazines.
Scissors.
Glue.
Felt pens.
Large sheet of paper.
Newspaper.
Use a large working table and chairs around it.

Procedure

Explain the exercise as follows:
'We are going to make a collage using magazine pictures.'

'First, however, we have to choose a theme. Does anyone have any suggestions?' (You can give a few examples for possible themes, e.g. leisure-time, anger, family life, things I have enjoyed.)	This part of the exercise requires a group decision which is the first first step toward cohesion.

'Then I would like you to go through the magazines and find pictures or examples of that theme. Cut the pictures out.'	This gives each person an opportunity for self-expression and personal interpretation of the theme.

Ask the first group member who appears restless to arrange the contributions for the collage on a sheet of background paper. Engage the next restless person to assist him in sticking them on.	Giving this job to the person who finds the first part of the exercise difficult, perhaps due to anxiety or poor concentration, will provide him with a constructive outlet for his restlessness.[1]

Make sure each group member is represented by at least one contribution.	This ensures that the collage is a group product and represents each person's involvement in the task (e.g. his feelings, his past experiences, his ideas as they relate to the theme, etc.).

'When the collage is complete we will discuss the theme and the pictures that each of us chose.' Suggest that the group hang the collage up.	To promote discussion amongst the participants. Once hung, the collage is a visual display of the group's ability to work together.

Discussion topics
- How easy or difficult was it to find pictures that related to the theme?
- Why did each person choose his particular pictures?
- What were your feelings about the theme?
- How did the group work together and what part did each person play in the task?

Your variations

---

1. Arranging and pasting the pictures could also be a group task requiring cooperation, compromise, decision-making and imagination on everyone's part.

Allow about 30 minutes
Group size: 8–12 young adults

Caboose (warm-up)

This is an exercise involving physical contact, cooperation and the chance to experience a protected versus a protective role.

Recommended for these problems

Model of Human Occupation
Vol.   – limited self-concept
Perf.   – depression as indicated by psychomotor retardation
         – impairment of interpersonal communication skills as indicated by social isolation

Life-style Performance Model
Sens/mo. – limited gross motor coordination
Psyc.   – lowered ability to assess personal skills
         – depression
Intp.   – limited social interaction

Stage of group development

This can be used as a warm-up exercise but it should be done with a group that has developed some degree of trust. It is useful to introduce when some of the group members are becoming restless.

Synopsis

In form, this exercise is a variant of Dodgeball. The players encircle two group members, one of whom shields the other. The players throw the ball and attempt to hit the protected person below the knee.

Materials and equipment

A large, soft ball, e.g. foam or 'nerf' ball.[1]
Use a large room.

Procedure

Invite the group to form a circle.	The act of forming a circle requires cooperation amongst the members, which may in turn stimulate greater awareness of themselves and others.
Explain the exercise as follows: 'We are going to play a variation of Dodgeball.'	To aid in comprehension by relating new experiences to familiar past experiences.
'Instead of one, there will be two people in the centre of the circle.'	To provide a comfort to those people who dislike being the target of attention.

1. Many people are afraid of being hit by a thrown ball: a soft ball is less anxiety-provoking.

'We will try to tag the first person (whom we will call *It*) with the ball while the second person (whom we will call the *Shield*) will try to deflect the ball and thereby protect his partner.'[2]

To give an opportunity for each person to play one of two roles: firstly, the guardian which is a protective role and secondly, the guarded which is a dependent role.

Once the individual has played a protective role and found it quite easy he may have more confidence in his protector when he is *It*.

'When *It* is successfully tagged he is out. (To tag successfully the ball must hit *It* below the knees.) Then the *Shield* becomes *It* and the person who threw the ball becomes the *Shield*.'

The individual is rewarded for teamwork and coordination by taking on the responsible role of protector. This is in contrast to regular Dodgeball where there is no reward other than remaining on the team.

As soon as any member of the group shows signs of restlessness, either change to another game or stop for a discussion.

Discussion topics
– What were the similarities and differences between the two roles?
– Did you enjoy working as a team?
– How do you feel after doing this physical exercise?

Your variations

2. It is much more difficult to tag in this manner. Team cooperation is needed to pass the ball quickly between players in order to catch the unprotected *It* from behind. This has the effect of increasing concentration, interaction and cooperation between the individual group members.

Compliments

Allow 1 hour
Group size: 8 adults/6 children

This is an exercise concerned with increasing awareness both of other people and oneself. It exercises the skills of perception, observation and memory.

Recommended for these problems

Model of Human Occupation
Vol. – decreased belief in personal effectiveness
– limited self-concept
– lack of interest in others as shown by passivity
– decreased expectations of success
Perf. – decreased concentration as indicated by forgetfulness
– impairment of interpersonal communication skills as indicated by social isolation

Life-style Performance Model
Cog. – diminished retention and recall
Psyc. – loss of self-esteem
– lowered ability to assess personal skills
Interp. – decreased interest in others
– limited social interaction

Stage of group development

This exercise is suitable for a group in which the members know one another fairly well but do not give one another support. It is good for a group with low morale.[1]

Synopsis

Each individual writes down everything he can remember about a group member who is out of sight. This person returns to the group and these observations are then shared and discussed.

Materials and equipment

Sheets of paper.
Pencils.

---

1. Because the comments will, for the most part, be constructive and encouraging and result in the increased confidence and self-esteem of the participants. It should also be used in groups where the participants are very isolated, since it will encourage them to make some degree of contact with each other. This should result in an increased awareness of each other and more group cohesion.

Procedure

Invite the group members to sit in a small circle on the floor.	This assists a sense of cohesion within the group and a relaxed atmosphere.
Ask them to pass around the paper and pencils, keeping one of each for themselves.	This encourages a decision to participate actively.
Explain the exercise as follows: 'One person will volunteer to leave the room.'	This allows each individual to decide whether he wishes to expose himself to comments from other people.
'While he is away, the remainder of the group will each make a list of the things[2] they can remember about him (e.g. physical appearance, clothing, likes or dislikes, personal strengths, etc.).	This encourages increased awareness of other people. It means one has to think carefully about the person and recall facts, events, feelings, etc. pertaining to him.
'When everyone has written all they can, the person outside the room will return and join the circle.'	
Each participant will then be invited to read out what he has written down.	This promotes direct verbal comment from one person to another. It provides an opportunity to give and receive positive observations which increase self-confidence.
Discussion should be encouraged.[3]	This encourages comparison of perceptions and an opportunity to clarify the feedback.

Discussion topics
  – Do the comments compare or contrast with how each person sees himself?
  – Why are the comments and observations of others important?
  – In what situations does one normally receive comments about oneself from other people?
  – How does each person deal with the comments?

Your variations

---

2. This requirement can be made more specific, e.g. 'Write down all the problems that you remember he has.' At the same time, the person absent might list what he considers his problems to be. This would promote discussion, comparing and contrasting what the group see as problems and what the individual sees.
3. This exercise can be followed by a discussion of the types of things observed. It often happens that as the exercise progresses, the comments change from concrete observations of clothing, etc. to more abstract recollections of personality.

Friendship collage

Allow 1 hour
Group size: 8 adults/6 children

(Adapted from Stalker.[1])

This projective exercise encourages individuals to assess personal qualities found in themselves and others.

Recommended for these problems	**Model of Human Occupation**
	Vol. – limited self-concept
	– decreased belief in personal effectiveness.
	Hab. – role loss as indicated by lack of identity
	Perf. – impairment of interpersonal communication skills as indicated by social isolation
	Life-style Performance Model
	Psyc. – loss of self-esteem
	– lowered ability to assess personal skills
	Intp. – limited social interaction
	– withdrawal from reciprocal interpersonal relationships
Stage of group development	This exercise should be used with a group who have worked together for a few sessions and are beginning to trust one another.
Synopsis	Group members describe the qualities they like in a good friend. Then they draw a picture of themselves and add some descriptive words which describe some of their own friendly qualities.
Materials and equipment	2 large sheets of white paper. Felt pens or wax crayons or magazines, scissors and glue. Large comfortable room with or without a table and chairs.

Procedure

Ask everyone to sit in circle on the floor or around a table.	To physically unite the group.
Explain the exercise: 'Today we are going to discuss friendship – what is it that makes for a good friendship between two or more people and what are some of the characteristics each one of us have which make us able to be a good friend to someone else.'	It is important to explain the exercise so that group members know what will be expected of them. This relieves anxiety.

'Let's start by identifying the personality characteristics that we look for in a good friend.'

'Is there anyone who would like to be the secretary and make a list of all the suggestions?' Give this person a piece of paper and felt pen.	This provides an opportunity for someone who does not feel comfortable speaking up to take a responsible role.
Participants may say such words as nice, kind, good, honest, helpful, generous, enthusiastic, loyal, listens well, keeps secrets, etc. As group leader you may have to encourage the group members to come up with descriptive words by giving examples of friendly acts and assisting them to find the right words to describe it.	
When there are no more ideas forthcoming, suggest that the secretary post the list up on the wall where everyone can see it.	This will provide a reminder for those who are having difficulty remembering.
Place the second large sheet of paper in the middle of the group.	To re-focus the group.
Say, 'Now draw a simple picture of yourself, as part of this group. Help yourself to felt pens, wax crayons, magazines, etc.'	Each person has an opportunity to draw or cut out a picture of how they see themselves.
It may be more appropriate to ask members to find a picture of a person in a magazine to represent them and glue it on the paper.	Using ready-made pictures from magazines accomodates a wide range of artistic skills.
Ask, 'Does anyone need more time?'	To give those who are not finished the responsibility for informing the group how much more time they need.
'Now somewhere close to your drawing and in a cartoon bubble write some qualities that you possess that make you a good friend.'	This provides an opportunity to assess and acknowledge some personal strengths.
As group leader you may want to give a definite number of words e.g. three or five. Remind the members that they can refer to the list that was generated earlier for ideas. If anyone is unable to do this, invite the group members to identify some of this individual's personal strengths.	To relieve anxiety and set a limit.

When the collage is completed invite each person to share these special qualities that they have identified.

This encourages each person to reiterate some personal strengths and to receive compliments and support from the group.

A general discussion can follow if appropriate.

Discussion topics
- Why do the qualities we identified make for good and lasting friendship? Take each descriptive word and discuss separately.
- What personal qualities can destroy a friendship and why – e.g. mean, selfish, lying, complaining, unpunctual, dishonest, aggressive, interfering, interrupting, etc.? Generate a list and discuss each one.
- Can you be friends with your brothers and sisters? Are friendships between siblings the same as other friendships?
- How does a person communicate that he cares without using words? e.g. being punctual, making eye-contact, listening without interrupting, hugging, sitting close, smiling, etc.

Your variations

REFERENCES

1. Stalker, A. (1991) *Bridges to Competence, Activities for Theme-based Social Skills Groups.* Available from the Occupational Therapy Department, British Columbia's Children's Hospital, 4480 Oak St., Vancouver, B.C., V6H 3V4, Canada.

Gifts

Allow 30 minutes
Group size: 8 adults/6 children

This is a simple exercise which facilitates a deeper understanding of self and a positive interaction with each group member.

Recommended for these problems

Model of Human Occupation

Vol.
- limited self-concept
- loss of internal locus of control as indicated by difficulty differentiating feelings
- difficulty initiating social interaction
- decreased belief in self as indicated by low self-esteem

Hab.
- feelings of incompetence

Life-style Performance Model

Psyc.
- lowered ability to assess personal skills
- difficulty understanding and expressing feelings
- loss of self-esteem

Intp.
- limited interpersonal skills

Stage of group development

This exercise is most successful when it is done with a group in which the members have developed some interest in one another.

Synopsis

All the group members give imaginary gifts to one another. These are delivered in written form.[1]

Materials and equipment

Paper.
Pencils.
Use a room with table and chairs.

Procedure

Invite the group members to sit around the table; then hand out a sheet of paper and pencil to each person.

Give the following directions:
'Fold and tear your piece of paper so that you have the same number of pieces as there are people in the group.'

This step is useful to observe anyone with particular perceptual difficulties.

---

1. The exercise can be done verbally if the group members are well motivated and able to be spontaneous. It can also be used verbally as a welcoming or farewell gesture towards a specific group member.

'On each slip write a name and the gift, such as a specific wish, that you would like to give to that person.'
'Take time to think carefully about each person so that you can make your gifts appropriate, personal and different for each one of us.'

To provide an opportunity for making a positive gesture towards other people in an anonymous and unspoken way.

When most people have finished ask:
'Does anyone need more time?'

To give those who have not finished the responsibility of informing the group when they are finished.

When everyone is ready ask them to give their slips of paper to the appropriate people.

Each person is then invited to read out his collection of gifts.

The gifts received not only give a measure of the impression we make on others, but also tend to be a joyful collection that enhances the self-concept.

He is asked not to identify the person who gave him each gift.

This ensures that the gift remains a personal and private gesture between two individuals.

Discussion topics – Is it difficult to give or receive compliments?
– How does each person feel about his collection of gifts? Were there any surprises?

Your variations

Guided exploring

Allow 20–30 minutes
Group size: 12 adults

This is an exercise to increase trust and sensory awareness.[1]

Recommended for these problems

Model of Human Occupation

Vol.   – feelings of powerlessness over personal actions resulting in apathy
       – impairment of interpersonal communication skills as indicated by:
           difficulty trusting people
           social isolation
Perf. – difficulty interpreting sensory cues

Life-style Performance Model

Sens/mo. – limited tactile discrimination
Psyc.   – apathy
Intp.   – limited capacity for trust
          – limited social interaction

Stage of group development

This exercise is appropriate to use with a group whose members are acquainted but are having difficulty trusting one another.

Synopsis

In pairs, group members take turns leading and being led about a room, with their eyes closed. The person is guided to explore the space and identify objects without the use of vision.

Materials and equipment

None.
Use a familiar room which has furniture in it.

Procedure

Invite the group members to choose a partner with whom they feel comfortable.	To initiate social interaction and decision-making.
Explain the exercise as follows: 'Will each pair decide between them who is to be the leader and who is to be guided.'	To encourage cooperative interaction.

---

1. The exercise is suitable for *videotaping*. The replay can be used to show the relationships between partners. The tape will also record the subtle nonverbal reactions of participants which can be used as a basis for discussion.

'Will the one to be guided close his eyes and try to keep them closed throughout the exercise.'	This will provide him with the experience of placing himself in the care of another person.
'Meanwhile, the leader will gently guide his partner around the room making sure that he does not hurt himself.'	To encourage a sense of responsibility and protectiveness towards another person. To give some degree of physical contact.
Address the leaders: 'When you feel he trusts you …'	To help develop awareness of how his partner is feeling as expressed by body movements.
'take his hand and guide it toward objects in the room, inviting him to identify them through his sense of touch.'	To increase the capacity for accurately perceiving things using senses other than sight, and to provide an opportunity for enjoying the world in this way.
'Do this for 5 minutes and then change roles.' (The time limit is arbitrary, but should be long enough to enable the person with closed eyes to become relaxed and at ease, and short enough to prevent him becoming bored.)	
When this part of the exercise is over, invite the group members to sit in a circle and share their feelings about the experience, first sharing with partners and then with the rest of the group.	To reunite the group in a physical manner.

Discussion topics
- Did you feel more comfortable leading or being led?
- What was it like to touch objects? What feelings did this arouse?
- Were you able to place your trust in another person?
- Were you afraid of bumping into objects and hurting yourself?
- How did you react?
- Did you experience the space differently with your eyes closed?
- Did you sense how your partner was feeling?
- Does being sensitive to how other people are feeling help one's relationships?

Your variations

Happiness

Allow 1 hour
Group size: 8 adults/6 children

This exercise uses reminiscing to help a person feel positive about himself.

Recommended for these problems

Model of Human Occupation

Vol.
  – depression as indicated by feelings of hopelessness or aimlessness
  – loss of sense of identity
  – decreased belief in self as indicated by loss of self-esteem

Hab.
  – feelings of incompetence
  – loss of valued roles

Perf.
  – impairment of interpersonal communication skills as indicated by social anxiety and isolation

Life-style Performance Model

Psyc.
  – depression
  – feelings of anxiety
  – loss of self-esteem

Intp.
  – limited social interaction

Stage of group development

This exercise can be used at any stage of group cohesion.

Synopsis

In this exercise each person relaxes and recalls a pleasant experience, then reproduces that vision on paper and shares the images which he has remembered.

Materials and equipment

White paper.
Felt pens, crayons.
Chairs around a table

Procedure

Ask the group members, seated around a table, to assume a position that is comfortable and relaxed.
Encourage them to uncross their arms, legs, or feet and let their hands lie loosely but supported. Ask them to close their eyes and take a deep breath and then let it out.

To avoid distraction from external stimuli and assist each person to become still, both physically and mentally – images will occur more easily in this state.

Give the following instructions:

'Remember a time when you felt warm and content; a time long ago or more recently when you had a sense that life was good,[1] that you were in tune with the people and things around you and you felt peaceful, confident and completely happy.' (Pause)	To help each person relax completely and move into a deeper state of consciousness where positive feelings can emerge.
'Remember the details of the place where you felt this way. Look around you and see the colours, the sounds, the smells … remember who was with you at that time.'	To help the individual sharpen the image he is experiencing.
'I will stop speaking now for a few minutes so that you can recall and enjoy that place.'	Silence is essential now to allow personal recall.
After a few minutes invite them to open their eyes and return to the present when they feel ready.	To help them to return to the present time without startling them.
Ask them to take a sheet of paper and some colours[2] and reproduce the place they have just seen.[3]	
Explain that artistic quality is not important, and that any way they draw their time of great happiness will be just as it should be, since no one else can know what they have just seen.	To relieve the anxiety aroused by the fear of pictorial expression through art.
Invite each member in turn to share his experience. Encourage the group to enjoy that experience with him through questions.	A sense of well-being is derived this way, both personally and vicariously.
Close the group by explaining that at present they are experiencing a difficult time, that much effort is spent looking at problems, but it is useful to recall past happiness and past strengths to be able to 'recharge the batteries' and to derive the energy to face and solve these problems.	To focus the individuals, in closing, on the positive aspects of this exercise, especially for those members who become depressed when comparing their emotional state now with the past.

Your variations

1. This exercise makes it possible for depressed people to experience briefly a sense of well being. It may be necessary for them to search back to their childhood in order to find it.
2. If there is much anxiety over art therapy, keep these materials initially on a separate table out of sight but readily available when needed to eliminate any needless delay between the experience and the depiction of it.
3. A variation of this exercise is to show them a mandala and ask them to describe the experience by drawing one, depicting their impressions in colour and abstract form, using the circle's outer limits to contain that memory.

How I feel today

Allow 1 hour
Group size: 8 adults/6 children

This is an exercise in self-awareness that focuses on feelings and their effect on communication.

Recommended for these problems	**Model of Human Occupation**	
	Vol.	– inability to make decisions
		– limited self-concept
		– loss of internal locus of control as indicated by difficulty differentiating feelings
	Perf.	– impairment of interpersonal communication skills as indicated by social isolation
	Life-style Performance Model	
	Psyc.	– lowered ability to assess personal skills
		– difficulty understanding and expressing feelings
	Intp.	– limited social interaction

Stage of group development This exercise succeeds when some degree of trust has developed between the members.

Synopsis In this simple projective technique, the group members relax and determine how they are feeling. They depict this in an image on paper, then discuss it with the rest of the group.

Materials and equipment White paper.
Coloured felt pens, crayons.
Pencils.
Chairs around a table.

Procedure

Ask the group members to find a comfortable position on their chairs, with arms and legs uncrossed and hands placed loosely on their laps.	To reduce all external stimuli so as to facilitate concentration – images will occur more easily in this state.
Suggest that each person close his eyes and try to relax completely. Then ask the group to recall their predominant feeling during that day and how this feeling has shown itself in their interactions with others.	By transforming the feeling state into a visual image, each person is able to look at it in greater detail and some of the reasons for that feeling usually emerge.

Then ask them to open their eyes and when they are ready put the feeling down on paper in some sort of symbolic way. Explain that it can be expressed as a design, an animal or object, etc. A variation of this is to ask them to shape clay to symbolize how they feel.

To offer a nonverbal manner in which to express feelings.

When everyone has finished ask group members to talk about their drawings if they wish.

To help the person see more clearly that his emotional state does make a difference to others, and to see that it may cause some of the difficulties he has had in relating to others.

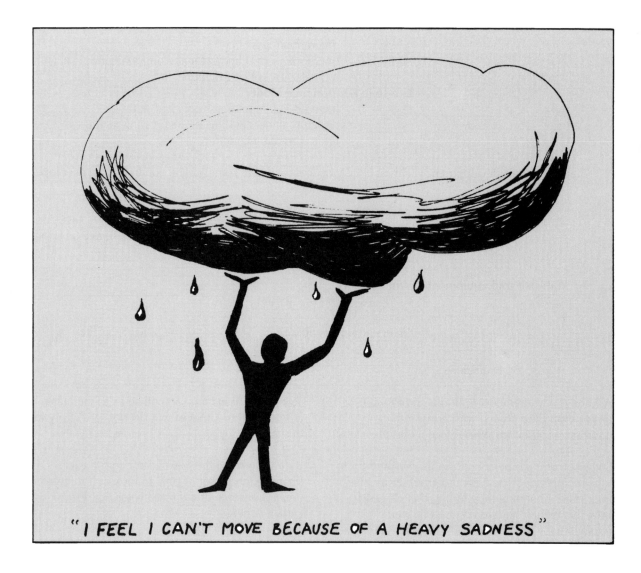

"I FEEL I CAN'T MOVE BECAUSE OF A HEAVY SADNESS"

Discussion topics
  – How this feeling affected the way he related to other people around him.
  – If he thought others perceived how he was feeling.
  – If people or events altered his feeling in any way.
  – Do our feelings affect the way we get along with our family, friends and our daily life?
  – In what different ways can we express our feelings? Explore the difference between verbal and nonverbal expression.

Your variations

Life-sized portrait

Allow 1 hour
Group size: 8 adults/6 children

This is a *projective technique* in self-awareness and expression of feelings.

Recommended for these problems

Model of Human Occupation
Vol.
  – limited self-concept
  – distorted body image
  – loss of internal locus of control as indicated by difficulty differentiating feelings

Life-style Performance Model
Sens/mo. – distorted body image
Psyc.   – lowered ability to assess personal skills
         – difficulty understanding and expressing feelings

Stage of group development

The exercise is only appropriate when the group members have developed some degree of trust for one another.

Synopsis

Each person has his body outlined on a large sheet of paper. He paints within the outline to show how he is feeling.

Materials and equipment

Roll of 1 m wide paper.
Watercolour paints.
Large paint brushes (e.g. 2.5 cm decorator brushes).[1]
Water containers.
Water.
Overalls.
Felt pens.
Masking tape.
Use a large room with a sink unit in it and preferably no other furniture.[2]

Procedure

Instruct each person as follows:
'Tear off a sheet of paper which is taller than yourself.'

The gross movement occurring tends to be tension reducing, which helps to prepare the person for freer movements when he is painting. An estimation of his own height is required.

---

1. To promote more spontaneity, provide larger paint brushes and reduce the time allotted for the portrait painting. This will also give additional time for discussion.
2. To promote a sense of responsibility, ask some or all of the group members to collect and return the materials needed, prepare the room and assist the less able participants.

'Place this sheet of paper on the floor and lie on it, finding the position in which you are most comfortable and entirely relaxed.'	This encourages each person to relax and be calm. The therapist can assess each person's ability to follow the instructions.
'Let me know when you are comfortable.' Using a felt pen, draw around the first person who says he is comfortable, making an outline of his body.	To encourage self-awareness and decision-making.
Invite this person to take the marker and draw around another person who says he is ready, and so on until each person has been outlined.[3]	This task requires coordination and physical contact with another person. It may also increase awareness of body image through the sense of touch.
Continue with the following instructions: 'Show how you feel, right now, by painting inside your own outline.'	This allows each person to express how he is feeling, graphically, and encourages him to search and identify the emotions inside him.
'Use different colours for the different feelings you are experiencing.'	So that more than one feeling may be expressed.
'Do *not* depict the clothes you are wearing.' 'Try to be finished in 15 minutes.'	To discourage a concrete response. This is to encourage uninhibited expression by each person and aid in the therapist's assessment of the ability to complete a task within a given time. The therapist should also observe such aspects as colour choice, manner of application and interaction.
When the time allowance is up invite each person to explain the feelings he has portrayed in his painting (see illustration).	To assist the person to communicate his feelings verbally using the nonverbal material as a reference.
Encourage discussion about the portraits by the group.	This is to develop awareness of other people and their feelings, and encourage the participants to check the accuracy of their perceptions.

Discussion topics
– How can colour be used to express feelings?
– Do our internal feelings change or are they always the same?
– If they change, what makes that happen?
– In what other ways can we express our feelings?
– Do we make our feelings known even when we are not speaking and if so, how?

Your variations

---

3. If the group is large or the attention span of the members short, ask them to choose a partner and outline each other. This will ensure that the outlining part of the activity takes a shorter period of time.

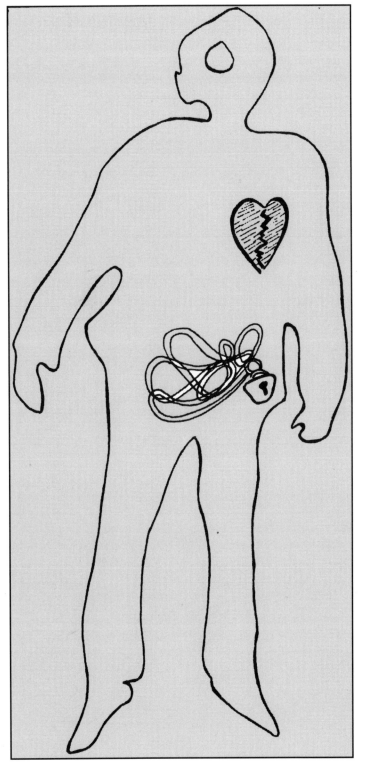

"THIS SHOWS A LARGE EMPTY AREA IN MY HEAD, AND MY STOMACH IS TIED UP IN KNOTS, PADLOCKED BUT I CAN'T FIND THE KEY ... I FEEL DETACHED FROM MY FAMILY ... I FEEL I DO EVERYTHING IN A MECHANICAL WAY"

SELF-PORTRAIT

Masks

Allow 1 hour
Group size: 8 adults/6 children

This exercise in self-awareness focuses on how people's facial expression can mask true feelings.

Recommended for these problems

Model of Human Occupation
Vol. – loss of internal locus of control as indicated by:
  lack of insight
  difficulty differentiating and expressing feelings
Perf. – decreased social involvement

Life-style Performance Model
Psyc. – difficulty understanding and expressing feelings
  – lowered ability to assess personal skills
Intp. – withdrawal from reciprocal interpersonal relationships

Stage of group development

This exercise is suitable to use with a group that has worked together for a few sessions and whose members are beginning to trust one another.

Synopsis

Each person is asked to draw his own face twice, firstly in terms of how others see it, and secondly in terms of how he actually feels inside. The group then discuss the resulting pictures.

Materials and equipment

Sheets of moderately stiff paper, about 20 cm × 28 cm.
Felt pens (wide colour range).
Pencils.
Room with table and chairs.

Procedure

Invite the group members to sit around the table …	To promote a sense of group cohesion and a purposeful atmosphere.
and each to take two sheets of paper.	This encourages each person to make the decision whether he will participate in the exercise or not.
Place the felt pens in the centre of the table.	To encourage cooperative interaction while working.
Give the following instructions: 'On one of your pieces of paper draw a picture of your face which shows how you think it appears to other people. Title this *How I appear to others*.'	To assist each person to be objective with regard to his outward appearance.

When everyone has finished, continue with the second part of the exercise.

'Now, thinking carefully of how you feel inside, draw another picture of your face (using the second piece of paper) to show how you actually feel. Title this *How I actually feel.*'	To increase the awareness of feelings at a particular point in time and to assist differentiation between outward and inward expression of them. To aid the therapist's assessment of each person's mental state.
When everyone has finished both parts of the exercise, invite each person to show the group his two drawings and to explain them.	To provide each person with an opportunity to explain his own drawings and promote increased awareness amongst everyone of how facial expression can be used to mask true feelings.
Encourage the group members to discuss any ideas or reactions they may have.	To help them become aware of the importance of nonverbal communication.
Also, invite them to become more aware of how often they notice themselves and others using their *mask* rather than expressing their real feelings.	This may promote greater self-awareness and encourage the giving and receiving of personal comments.
Note: Displaying the *masks* on the walls of the group's room can act as a reminder to them of the exercise.	

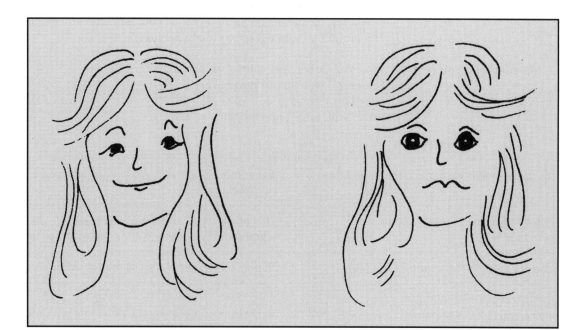

HOW I APPEAR   HOW I ACTUALLY FEEL

Discussion topics
- What might cause a person to hide feelings?
- What are the effects upon oneself and others of masking one's feelings?
- Do you feel you understand others better once you have heard how they actually feel?

Your variations

Allow 30 minutes
Group size: 8 adults/6 children

Memory game

The purpose of this exercise is to improve an individual's perception and memory, particularly in relation to objects.

Recommended for these problems

Model of Human Occupation
Vol.   – loss of internal locus of control as indicated by lack of interaction with the environment
Perf.   – decreased concentration as indicated by forgetfulness
Life-style Performance Model
Cog.   – short attention span
        – diminished retention and recall
Psyc.   – apathy
        – difficulty sustaining contact with external stimuli

Stage of group development

This is an excellent exercise to use with a group who are not physically active and have a short attention span.

Synopsis

A tray of common objects is presented for the participants to look at. After a short period of time, this tray is removed from sight. The players attempt to recall as many of the objects as they can.

Materials and equipment

Tray with cover.
Small common objects.
Pencils.
Paper.
Room with table and chairs.

Procedure

Invite the participants to sit around the table and each take a pencil and paper.[1]	To provide an opportunity for each person to be physically involved in the exercise.
Explain the game as follows: 'I shall place a tray with 10 objects on it, in the middle of the table.'[2]	
The therapist may wish to invite some of the players to put together their own trays of objects and in turn present them to the group.	Provides an opportunity for the individual to use his initiative and also may assist the therapist in her assessment of him.
'You will have four minutes to look at the tray and memorize the objects.'	To encourage concentration, attention to detail and memorization.
'The tray will then be removed and each of you will write down as many of the objects as you can recall.'	To practise the skill of immediate recall.
'I shall then bring back the tray for you to check your answers.'	To enable each person to measure his level of achievement privately.
In the discussion focus on different methods of recall, e.g visual, auditory, etc.	To help them transfer this skill into daily life, e.g. remembering names.

Discussion topics
- What way did you use to remember the objects? Did you remember what the objects looked like on the tray, group them according to use, colour, shape, size or recall them as a learned list?
- In what situations is a good memory important?

Your variations

---

1. This game can be played by individuals, pairs, or teams according to the needs of the participants. For example, if they are very isolated then have them play in twos or threes since this will necessitate the interaction of one person with another and the sharing of ideas.
2. The number of objects on the tray should be varied according to the mental state of the participants. It is better to start with a low number of objects and increase the number each time the game is played, so as to provide a sense of accomplishment and improvement amongst the participants. This may in turn increase their motivation. To provide a sense of involvement and responsibility, the therapist may wish to invite some of the players to put together their own trays of objects and in turn present them to the group. This provides an opportunity for the individual to use his initiative and also may assist the therapist in her assessment of him.

Now and the future

Allow 1 hour
Group size: 8 adults

This is an exercise which assists individuals to gain a deeper understanding of themselves and of each other.

Recommended for these problems

Model of Human Occupation
Vol.   – difficulty conceptualizing future events
           – decreased expectations of success
           – loss of internal locus of control as indicated by lack of insight
Hab.   – decreased motivation for behavioural change
           – role loss as indicated by lack of identity
Perf.   – deficiency in process skills affecting planning

Life-style Performance Model
Cog.   – difficulty making choices
           – limited motivation for behavioural change
Psyc.   – lowered ability to assess personal skills

Stage of group development

This exercise is best for a group that has developed some unity and in which the members have some interest in each other.

Synopsis

Each person compares his present situation with his desired future situation, depicting both of them in diagrammatic form.

Materials and equipment

White paper.
Pencils and erasers.
Felt pens.
Table and chairs.

Procedure

Invite everyone to sit around the table and help themselves to paper and pencils.	To initiate active participation.
Ask the group members to fold their paper in half (demonstrate with your own paper).	
Give the following instructions: 'On the left side of your piece of paper draw *how you are now*. That is, how you are feeling and what your present life situation is. Then, on the	To give the individual an opportunity to look at his present situation clearly and to project himself into a future, relieved of his present problems.

right side, draw *how you wish to be in the future.*
Draw diagrams and symbols to explain your
situation. Don't be artistic or draw a self-portrait.'

When most people are finished, ask, 'Does anyone need more time?'	To allow those people who either have much to say or who find the exercise difficult, to work at their own speed. They will take the responsibility for telling the group when they are ready.
When the group is ready, ask who would like to begin by explaining his drawings. If the discussion is awkward ask him to him to compare the two drawings and explain how he hopes to attain his desired future.	To stimulate some dynamic thoughts about life as he sees it and possible changes he can make.

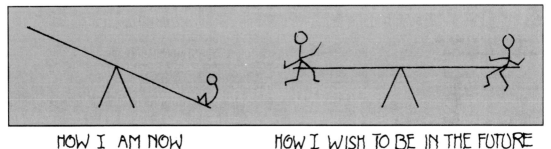

HOW I AM NOW   HOW I WISH TO BE IN THE FUTURE

Discussion topics   – Discuss methods of changing present situations.
– Discuss fear of the future (e.g. jobs and other commitments).
– What it is like to feel helpless about making decisions about your life?
– Discuss taking on responsibility for one's own life and its direction.

Your variations

Painting to music

Allow 1 hour
Group size: 8 adults/6 children

This is a *projective exercise* to assist self-expression.

Recommended for these problems

Model of Human Occupation
Vol.   – limited self-concept
          – loss of internal locus of control as indicated by difficulty differentiating feelings
Perf.   – difficulty expressing ideas due to limited interpersonal communication skills

Life-style Performance Model
Cog.   – difficulty expressing ideas
Psyc.   – lowered ability to assess personal skills
          – difficulty understanding and expressing feelings

Stage of group development
This exercise works well with a group of people who are acquainted with each other but need some means of expressing themselves in a group setting.

Synopsis
After listening to a piece of music, each person creates a painting to express the images or feelings that were evoked.

Materials and equipment
C.D.s or taped music (see Suggestions, below).
Tape deck or C.D. player.
Sheets of paper, at least 40 cm × 50 cm
Watercolour paints.
Paint brushes of assorted sizes.
Water containers.
Newspaper.
Overalls (optional).
Tables and chairs (optional).
Use a room with enough working space to promote a relaxed atmosphere.

Procedure

Invite everyone to sit in a circle, finding a really comfortable position.	To assist each person to listen attentively to the music.

Explain the exercise as follows:
'I am going to play a short extract of music through twice.'[1]

Clear, concise instructions tend to reassure those who are fearful of new experiences.

'As you listen to it, try to be aware of what it makes you think of and how it makes you feel. Then collect some paint and paint brushes and express these feelings on paper.'

To encourage self-awareness and concentration.

'No doubt, we shall all experience the music differently; some of us may respond to the rhythm, others to the feelings or images aroused within ourselves.'

To give reassurance and encourage each person to feel safe enough to express his reactions, even if they are different from those of the person next to him.
The therapist should observe how each person reacts.

'Wait until you feel ready to start.'

To enable reluctant participants to join in later on.[2]

'Later there will be an opportunity for each person to explain his painting if he so wishes.'[3]

This will provide an opportunity for each person to share his feelings with the others.

Encourage discussion by sharing one's own reactions and assisting group members to share theirs.

To increase awareness of one's self and others, and to encourage the giving and receiving of comments.

Suggestions for 'Painting to music'

Musical selections suitable for stimulating a variety of emotional responses

Adagio Opus 11 (1)	Samuel Barber
Air on a G String	Bach
Ave Maria	Schubert
Ecossaises	Beethoven
Gymnopedies 1 or 3	Eric Satie
Latin American Symphonette	Morton Gould
Moonlight Sonata: (first movement)	Beethoven

---

1. It is not necessary to identify the music until the end of the exercise. This should encourage the expression of spontaneous rather than preconceived ideas and feelings.
2. With some groups it may be advisable to set a time limit. Do not be too concerned if someone does not wish to participate – it is likely he/she will when he/she sees the others involved and at ease.
3. Our experience with this exercise has shown that: it tends to provide the very quiet person with an opportunity to express himself; the underlying feelings evoked in people are often similar, although their symbolic portrayal of the feelings may be different; the most withdrawn people are often the most perceptive.

Peer Gynt Suite No. 1:	
(Hall of the Mountain King)	Grieg
Piano Concerto No. 4 in G Major	
(first movement bars 1–29)	Beethoven
Rite of Spring (Part 1 'Adoration of the Earth')	Stravinsky
Scheherezade Suite: (first movement)	Rimsky-Korsakov
Scherzo No. 1 in B Minor, Opus 20	Chopin
Slavonic Dance No. 2	Dvorak
Symphony No. 5 in C Minor: (first movement)	Beethoven
The Four Seasons, Opus 8 nos. 1–4	Antonio Vivaldi
The Sorcerer's Apprentice	Dukas
William Tell Overture: (finale)	Rossini
Violin Concerto in D Major:	
(second movement bars 1–20)	Mozart
Xerxes (Largo)	Handel

Musical selections suitable for stimulating the imagination	*Night on the Bare Mountain*	Mussorgsky
	Dance of the Hours	Ponchielli
	Finlandia, Opus 26	Sibelius
	Nutcracker Suite	Tchaikovsky
	Pictures at an Exhibition	Mussorgsky
	Romeo and Juliet Overture	Tchaikovsky
	Symphony No. 6 in F Major ('Pastoral'), Opus 68	Beethoven
	The Planets, Opus 32	Gustav Holst
	The Vltava (Moldau)	Smetana
	Peter and the Wolf	Prokofiev

Discussion topics

– How did the music make you feel?
– Was painting a good way to express the feelings?
– Did the music suggest particular images to you?
– Do these images mean anything specific to you?

Perceptions

Allow 1 hour
Group size: 8 adults/6 children

This is a *projective technique* which uses diagrams to help members verbalize how they perceive themselves and how that may differ from the image they present to others.

Recommended for these problems

Model of Human Occupation

Vol.   – decreased motivation for behavioural change
       – decreased belief in self as indicated by low self-esteem
       – limited self-concept
       – decreased expectations of success
Hab.   – loss of identity as indicated by role imbalance
Perf.   – deficiency in process skills as indicated by difficulty planning

Life-style Performance Model

Cog.   – limited motivation for behavioural change
Psyc.   – loss of self-esteem
       – lowered ability to assess personal skills

Stage of group development

Use this exercise with group members who have formed some bonds of trust and are willing to share feelings with each other.

Synopsis

Three drawings are made by each person to contrast outward appearances with personal identity and to help suggest ways of changing.

Materials and equipment

Pencils with erasers.
White paper.
Table and chairs.

Procedure

Hand out a sheet of paper and pencil to each person.

Ask them to fold their sheet of paper into thirds. Demonstrate with your own paper.

At this point the therapist can assess which members have difficulty following directions.

Explain the exercise as follows:
'Label the first third of your paper *How others see me*, the middle third *How I see myself*, and the final third *How I would like to be seen*.'

'Now draw diagrams and symbols to depict yourself in each of the three areas.'

Using symbols rather than words may release feelings from below the conscious and, therefore, censorable level.

When most people seem to have finished, ask, 'Does anyone need more time?'

To give those who are not ready the responsibility for informing the group when they are finished.

When everyone has completed the exercise, ask each person to explain his set of diagrams to the group.

Encourage the group members to respond honestly when each person is discussing the category *How others see me*. Be prepared to help each person handle realistic comments. Encourage the group members to be constructive with any critical feedback they may give.

This gives each person an opportunity to see if his perceptions about how others view him are correct.

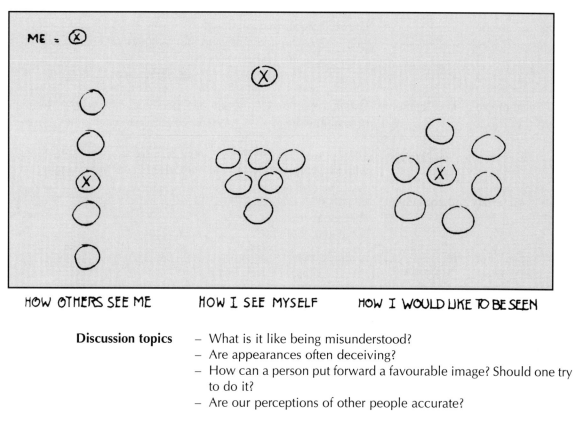

HOW OTHERS SEE ME   HOW I SEE MYSELF   HOW I WOULD LIKE TO BE SEEN

Discussion topics   – What is it like being misunderstood?
– Are appearances often deceiving?
– How can a person put forward a favourable image? Should one try to do it?
– Are our perceptions of other people accurate?

Your variations

<table>
<tr><td>Allow 1 hour
Group size: 10 adults/6 children</td><td># Personal symbols
(Created by Lily Jaffe, ATR, Vancouver, Canada.)</td></tr>
</table>

This exercise is a *projective technique* through which a person is able to see more clearly some of the basic beliefs that he holds about himself.

Recommended for these problems	**Model of Human Occupation**
	Vol. — limited self-concept
	— decreased belief in personal effectiveness
	Perf. — difficulty initiating social interaction
	Life-style Performance Model
	Psyc. — loss of self-esteem
	— lowered ability to assess personal skills
	Intp. — limited interpersonal skills

Stage of group development   Because some self-disclosure is needed, this exercise is best done with individuals who have formed some degree of trust.

Synopsis   In this exercise, each person discovers, in a random pattern they create, personal symbols whose qualities they compare to their own personalities.[1]

Materials and equipment   White paper.
Coloured felt pens.
Chairs around a table.

Procedure

Invite the group members to help themselves to paper and felt pens. Suggest they choose a colour most relevant to their present mood.

To help alleviate anxiety by taking an active role in choosing to participate.

Give the following instructions:
'Imagine an ant wandering all over your sheet of paper; make a line that shows what sort of track he would make. Let him go aimlessly, doubling back on his path when you want him to, and fill the entire sheet of paper.'

---

1. A variation of this exercise is to use objects, e.g. stones, shells, flowers, etc., found either by the group at the start of the session or by the leader prior to the session. Individuals are asked to choose an object that they are attracted to, to handle that object, noticing colour, shape, texture, function, etc. and to list those qualities. The remainder of the exercise is the same as the above.

When all the members have completed this part ask them to survey this pattern by half closing their eyes, thus allowing familiar or unfamiliar shapes to evolve, e.g. faces, people, animals, things, etc.	To help them shift into a different state of awareness.
Encourage them not to worry if the object only slightly resembles something or is a part of something.	To help those who may have difficulty with such a loose association of their vague shapes with precise images.
Ask them now to: 'Use a colour to trace the outlines of these objects; to put eyes, a nose, a mouth, ears, hair, or a tail for easier identification as well as permit yourself to modify the outlines to make them more relevant to your image.'	To help them make a physical decision and commitment when identifying various shapes. To make identification of the shapes quicker when discussing them later with the group.
Then say: 'Now look at each shape that you have outlined and ask yourself – what qualities or characteristics does it have. List these on the back of the paper.'	
Invite a volunteer to identify his images.[2] When he talks about the qualities expressed in the drawing, suggest that he consider the possibility that some of these might apply to him.	To make it possible for the individual to choose whether or not he wants to identify with some or any of the qualities attributed to the image. He may in fact identify with more than he wished to reveal to the group.
Ask questions when the personal beliefs are unclear. Do not assume or interpret for them connections between the object and themselves.[3]	

Discussion topics
- Are we more attracted to things or people who have similar qualities to ourselves?
- People are often more intolerant of faults in others than they are of their own.
- Note the adjectives you frequently use to describe things and see if they reflect your current mood.

Your variations

---

2. In reviewing the group, it will become evident that each person expressed one or two basic beliefs about himself that will be keys to his relationship with others.
3. For example, if a depressed person outlines a shoe, he may say he always tried to fit into his father's shoes, i.e. take the same career as his father, rather than your interpretation that he felt downtrodden.

Security

Allow 1 hour
Group size: 8 adults

This is an exercise to help individuals identify factors that promote or inhibit a feeling of security.

Recommended for these problems

Model of Human Occupation
Vol.   – diminished sense of personal effectiveness
Hab.   – loss of identity as indicated by role imbalance
Perf.   – inability to problem-solve
         – impairment of interpersonal communication skills

Life-style Performance Model
Cog.   – difficulty problem-solving
Psyc.   – loss of self-reliance
Intp.   – limited social interaction

Stage of group development

This exercise is most effective and successful with a group in which the members show some degree of interest in each other.

Synopsis

Each person depicts diagrammatically factors that bring security and insecurity, using a circle format; then attitudinal changes are discussed.

Materials and equipment

White paper.
Pencils.
Chairs around a table.

Procedure

Discuss briefly the role security plays in both physical and mental well-being; its connection with stress, decision-making, and relationships.	To help individuals begin to look at the importance security plays in their lives.
Beforehand, draw a heavy black circle approximately 12 cm in diameter in the centre of a 21 × 27 cm page. Make enough copies for the group.	The circle is an unconscious symbol of security or wholeness.[1] Working inside it visually elicits feelings that are the subject of this exercise.
Distribute the paper and pencils, then describe the exercise as follows: 'Think about those things in your life that make you feel secure and that bring you a sense of stability. Write or draw these things, whether they are people, objects or ideas, inside the circle...	

Now recall those things that bring a feeling of uneasiness and insecurity and add those outside the circle.'

When everyone has completed his diagram, ask for a volunteer to share his with the group. As he describes both sets of factors, suggest that he consider any relationship between the two, for example, parenting can bring both security and insecurity.

To help some group members discover that factors causing insecurity can also bring security, depending on their attitude.

Discuss amongst the group any changes that can be suggested to move items to inside the circle.

To promote problem-solving.

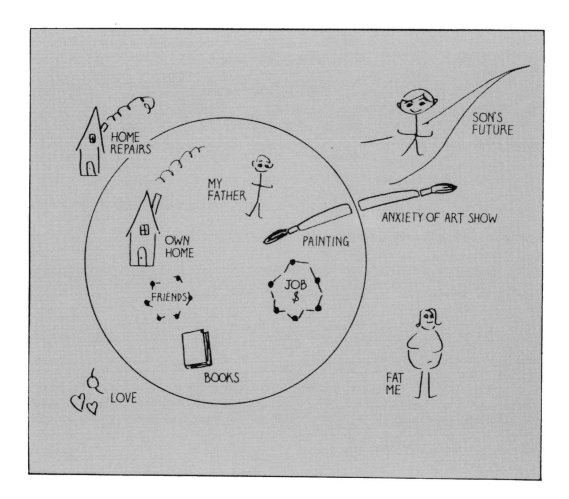

Discussion topics
- What are the differences or similarities between those things that make us feel secure and those that make us feel insecure?
- What things that make us feel secure do we have control over?
- Is the reverse true for those things that make us feel insecure?
- Who are the people that you can rely on?

Your variations

REFERENCES

1. Jung, Carl G. (1968) *Man and his symbols*, p. 240. New York: Doubleday and Co.

Allow 1 hour or more
Group size: 8 adults

Self-portrait collage

This is a *projective technique* in self-awareness and self-expression.

Recommended for these problems	**Model of Human Occupation**

Model of Human Occupation

Vol.   – loss of internal locus of control as indicated by difficulty differentiating feelings
      – limited self-concept

Hab.   – role imbalance

Perf.   – impairment of interpersonal communication skills as indicated by social isolation
      – limited task-orientated skills

Life-style Performance Model

Psyc.   – difficulty understanding and expressing feelings
      – lowered ability to assess personal skills and limitations

Intp.   – limited social interaction

Stage of group development

This exercise is very appropriate to use with a group containing many new members.[1]

Synopsis

Each person makes a collage to illustrate his personality and life-style and then discusses his portrayed identity.

Materials and equipment

Sheets of paper approximately 60 cm × 90 cm, one for each person.
Wide selection of magazines.
Scissors.
Glue.
Use a room which has sufficient working space or tables for the number of participants.

Procedure

Explain the exercise as follows:
'We are going to make individual collages. Imagine that a friend wishes to know all about you, but you are unable to speak.'

A clear explanation is needed to allay fears of having to perform and perhaps be judged.

---

1. This is an excellent technique to use with patients who have recently arrived in hospital or any other treatment setting. During the course of the exercise the therapist can make a general assessment of each patient, while the patient uses the exercise to settle in. By recalling the familiar life away from hospital and sharing this with unfamiliar people the patient achieves some degree of comfort and personal identity.

'Make a poster that illustrates your personality and life-style, by selecting appropriate pictures from these magazines.'

Magazines offer a variety of pictures that can be selected to represent various aspects of a person's life. This accommodates a wide range of artistic skills.

'Try to include pictures that show some of the following things about you (your attitudes and interests, likes and dislikes, characteristics, family, friends, jobs, ambitions, feelings, problems, reasons for being in hospital and so on).
Be selective, because it is impossible to illustrate every aspect of yourself.'[2]

To increase self-awareness and encourage appropriate selection, discrimination and coordination of pictures from a wide range of possibilities.

'Here are the magazines and scissors. Let me know when you need the background paper.'

To promote active participation and stimulate interest at the beginning of the exercise.

'Let's complete the collage in 20 minutes.'

Providing a set time in which to complete the task encourages organization in working. It also helps the overactive person control his need to be all-inclusive.

Besides making her own poster, the therapist will clarify the task for those who don't understand and encourage everyone while they are working.

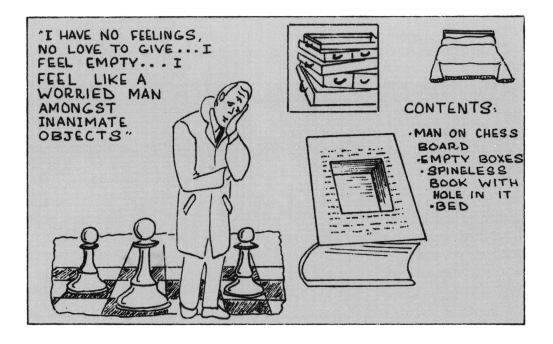

2. Analysis of the pictures selected will aid in the assessment of each person's perceptual and motor ability and mental state.

When the time is up ask, 'Does anyone need more time?'	To encourage each person to decide whether his collage is completed or not and to take responsibility for requesting more time.
When all are finished, invite each person to tell the group about his collage.	To provide an opportunity to share a brief portrait of their lives.
The therapist should share those parts of her collage that are appropriate.	This can provide a basis for social interaction.

Your variations

Support systems

Allow 1 hour
Group size: 8 adults/6 children

This is an exercise to help an individual to identify his existing support system and discuss its effectiveness.

Recommended for these problems

Model of Human Occupation

Vol.   – limited self-concept
Hab.   – inadequate support system
              – lack of identity due to role loss
Perf.   – difficulty initiating social interaction
              – decreased social involvement

Life-style Performance Model

Psyc.   – lowered ability to assess personal skills
Intp.   – withdrawal from reciprocal interpersonal relationships
              – limited interpersonal skills

Stage of group development

This exercise is most effective and successful with a group in which the members show some degree of interest in each other.

Synopsis

Each person makes a simple collage which depicts their support system. Individuals within the system are identified and their relationship to the key person is defined.

Materials and equipment

Magazines.
Glue.
Scissors.
Large sheets of paper.
Tables and chairs.

Procedure

Before handing out any of the materials explain the exercise as follows:	To catch the attention of the easily distracted individuals before they become engrossed in their magazines. To state the therapeutic purpose clearly before any deprecatory ideas associated with kindergarten materials emerge.

'Think about the people (friends and relations) who are important to you. The people to whom you turn when you are happy or sad, lonely or confused, for conversation or entertainment.'	To encourage awareness of various relationships in their lives.
'Look fairly quickly through the magazines and cut out pictures that represent these people. Do not concern yourself with likenesses.'	To allow the unconscious a chance to guide the choice and to discourage conscious reasoning.
'Find a picture to represent yourself as well.'	This choice may be quite revealing to both the participant and the therapist.
'Glue this picture on to the centre of your paper.' 'Then place your friends and relatives around you. Put those to whom you feel closest near or touching you on the paper and represent the distance you feel from the others by the distance they are placed from your picture in the centre.'	The spatial relationship used symbolically to represent an emotional relationship is a simple nonverbal tool that bypasses cognition.
Hand out the supplies and restate the instructions for anyone who had difficulty following them.	

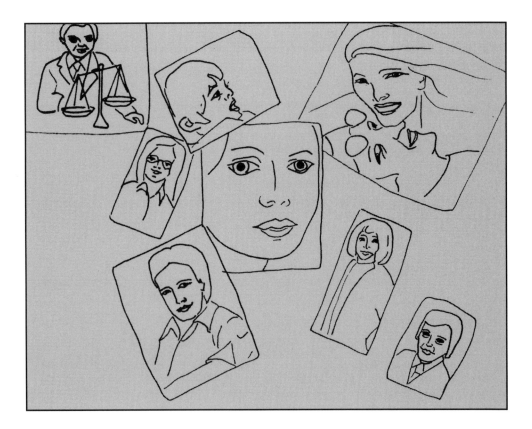

When most people have finished ask:
'Does anyone need more time?'

Allow time for the members and yourself to
explain their collages.
Encourage the group members to ask questions of
one another.

Discussion topics
    – The different roles family members play in our lives.
    – The tendency to rely on one person rather than a number of people.
    – The use of professionals and community facilities and services in a support system.

Your variations

Allow 1 hour
Group size: 8 adults

Time management

This is an exercise in time management, problem solving and awareness of one's lifestyle.

Recommended for these problems	**Model of Human Occupation**

Model of Human Occupation

Vol.   – loss of interèst in activities
Hab.   – role imbalance
          – loss of organizational skills
Perf.   – depression as indicated by social isolation
          – inability to problem-solve

Life-style Performance Model

Cog.   – difficulty problem-solving
Psyc.   – inability to manage time
Intp.   – limited interpersonal skills

Stage of group development   This exercise can be done with a group who do not know each other.

Synopsis   Each person calculates the various ways he spends his time in a 24-hour period then displays it on a pie graph.

Materials and equipment   Paper.
Pencils and erasers.
Coloured felt pens.
Chairs around a table.

Procedure

Beforehand, draw a circle, 16 cm in diameter in the bottom half of a 21 × 27 cm page. List above the circle on the left hand side: sleeping, eating and meal preparation, etc. Divide the circle into equal sections (see diagram.) Make enough copies of this for the group.

Introduce the topic of time management by talking about the importance of time planning, so as to achieve a balance of physical, emotional and spiritual parts of one's life.

Distribute the prepared sheets and pencils. Invite the participants to look at an average[1] 24-hour day and to calculate the time spent in the various activities listed at the top of the paper.

To help each person think in terms of total time spent (e.g. with hygiene) so that he will perceive the circle as a graph and not as a 24-hour clock where activities appear periodically throughout the day.

Then ask them to transfer this information onto the circle (divided into 24 equal wedges), blocking out time in sections, e.g. 8 hours of sleep would be blocked out using 8 wedges of the circle.
Suggest using a different colour for each activity as this makes it easier to see later. Move about the group assisting those who need more clarification.

To help those people who have difficulty seeing things graphically.

When everyone has finished, suggest that they share their information, beginning with a volunteer.

As each person describes his day invite the group members to ask questions and give suggestions. After everyone has had a turn, move into a period of open discussion.

To help, for example, the workaholic make time for relaxation or the depressed mother build in time for herself amid the endless household responsibilities.

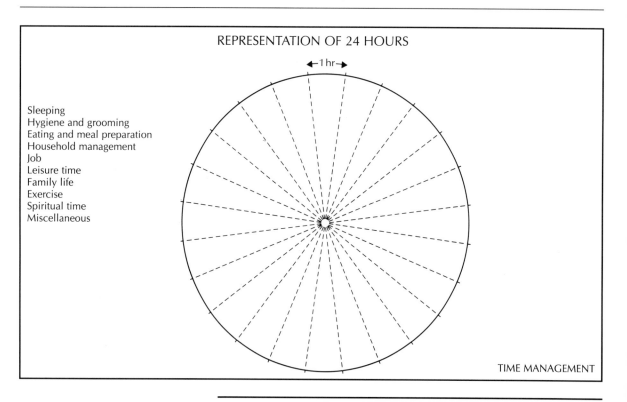

REPRESENTATION OF 24 HOURS

←1 hr→

Sleeping
Hygiene and grooming
Eating and meal preparation
Household management
Job
Leisure time
Family life
Exercise
Spiritual time
Miscellaneous

TIME MANAGEMENT

1. An average day outside hospital if they are currently inpatients.

Discussion topics
- What are the things that you would like to include in your day but don't have time for?
- Do you feel satisfied or dissatisfied with the amount of time you spend in any one category? Is it too much or too little?
- Can you suggest any alternatives so that you change what you don't like?
- How important is it to balance responsibilities with personal desires?
- In families where two parents are in fulltime work, how can the household responsibilities be shared around?

Your variations

Appendix A: sub-systems of the Model of Human Occupation

The exercises are listed according to the main sub-system which they address in the Model of Human Occupation:

VOLITION

Personal causation
Am I too close or too far away?
Caboose (warm-up)
Comment cards
Expressions
Guided exploring
Happiness
Life-sized portrait
Masks
Now and the future
Painting to music
Perceptions
Self-portrait collage
Simultaneous conversations

Values
Compliments
Friendship collage
Gifts
Personal symbols

Interests
Likes and dislikes
This is my life

HABITUATION

Roles
Support systems

Habits
Hand puppets
Time management

PERFORMANCE

Interpersonal
Charades
Continuing story
Cooperation
How I feel today
Introductions
Join me (warm-up)
Mirrors
Names (warm-up)

	Pass the ball (warm-up)
	People machine
	Persuasion
Process	Geography (warm-up)
	Monologue or dialogue
	Newspaper quiz
	Save yourself
	Security
	Soapbox
	Story-telling
	Theme collage
Perceptual motor	Action mime (warm-up)
	Exchanging chairs (warm-up)
	Getting acquainted with rhythm (warm-up)
	Magic box
	Memory game
	Movement and sound circle (warm-up)
	Mystery objects
	Name recall (warm-up)
	The matchbox is … ? (warm-up)
	Who stole the cookie from the cookie jar? (warm-up)
	Word circle (warm-up)

Appendix B: sub-systems of the Life-style Performance Model

The exercises are listed according to the main sub-system which they address in the Life-style Performance Model:

SENSORY MOTOR
Exchanging chairs (warm-up)
Getting acquainted with rhythm (warm-up)
Magic box
Movement and sound circle (warm-up)
Mystery objects
The matchbox is …? (warm-up)
Who stole the cookie from the cookie jar? (warm-up)

COGNITIVE
Action mime (warm-up)
Continuing story
Geography (warm-up)
Hand puppets
Memory game
Monologue or dialogue
Name recall (warm-up)
Newspaper quiz
Now and the future
Save yourself
Security
Soapbox
Story-telling
Theme collage
Time management
Word circle (warm-up)

PSYCHOLOGICAL
Comment cards
Compliments
Expressions
Friendship collage
Gifts
Happiness
Life-sized portrait
Likes and dislikes

Masks
Painting to music
Perceptions
Self-portrait collage
Personal symbols
Sort yourself out (warm-up)

INTERPERSONAL   Am I too close or too far away?
Caboose (warm-up)
Charades
Cooperation
Guided exploring
How I feel today
Introductions
Join me (warm-up)
Mirrors
Names (warm-up)
Pass the ball (warm-up)
People machine
Persuasion
Simultaneous conversations
Support systems
This is my life

Glossary of current psychiatric terms

This includes terms used in this handbook.

Accessible. 'Capable of being reached.'[1]

Acting out. 'Expressions of unconscious emotional conflicts or feelings of hostility or love in actions rather than words. The individual is not consciously aware of the meaning of such acts. May be harmful or in controlled situations, therapeutic (e.g. children's play therapy).'[2]

Activation. 'Stimulation of one organ-system by another; the term stimulation is generally reserved for external influences only.'[3]

Active therapist. 'Type of therapist who makes no effort to remain anonymous but is forceful and expresses his personality definitively in the therapy session.'[4]

Activity. 'In occupational therapy, any occupation or interest wherein participation requires exertion of energy.'[5] See also **Passivity**.

Activity group. 'In occupational therapy an activity in which several patients participate. Its chief value is its socializing effect upon the mentally ill patients who are asocial.'[6]

Activity, socializing. 'In therapy groups this term denotes the activity that brings an individual into interaction with other members of the group.'[7]

Affect. 'A person's emotional feeling tone and its outward manifestations. Affect and emotion are commonly used interchangeably.'[8]

Affect, blunted. 'A disturbance of affect manifested by dullness of externalized feeling tone. Observed in schizophrenia, it is one of that disorder's fundamental symptoms, according to Eugen Bleuler.'[9]

Aggression. 'A forceful physical, verbal or symbolic action. May be appropriate and self-protective, including healthful self-assertiveness, or inappropriate. Also may be directed outward toward the environment, as in explosive personality, or inward toward the self, as in depression.'[10]

Ambivalence. 'The coexistence of two opposing drives, desires, feelings, or emotions towards the same person, object, or goal. These may be conscious or partly conscious; or one side of the feelings may be unconscious. Example: love and hate toward the same person.[11]

Anger. 'A strong feeling of displeasure.'[12]

Antidepressant agents. 'These reduce the symptoms of major depression in which there is a significant loss of interest or pleasure in all facets of living, to such a degree that one's ability to function effectively is impaired.'[13]

Antipsychotic agents (neuroleptics). 'These drugs alleviate psychotic symptoms including cognitive-perceptual disorders (delusions, hallucinations), affective symptoms (apathy, withdrawal, depressions) and arousal symptoms (excitability, irritability, restlessness).'[14]

Anxiety. 'Apprehension, tension, or uneasiness that stems from anticipation of danger, the source of which is largely unknown or unrecognized. Primarily of intrapsychic origin, in distinction to fear, which is the emotional response to a consciously recognized and usually external threat or danger.' It 'may be regarded as pathological when present to such an extent as to interfere with effectiveness in living, achievement of desired goals or satisfactions, or reasonable emotional comfort.'[15]

Apathy. Lack of feelings or affect; 'lack of interest and emotional involvement in one's surroundings.'[16]

Aphasia. 'Loss of or impaired ability to speak, write or to understand the meaning of words, due to brain damage.'[17]

Apprehension. When used by psychiatrists, apprehension is almost invariably connected with the feeling of fear, anxiety, or dread. 'There is a tendency, however, to use more circumscribed expressions, such as anxiety, in place of such a general term as apprehension.' The term can also be used to describe 'the intellectual act or process by which a relatively simple object is understood, grasped, or brought before the mind.'[18]

Appropriate. 'Fitting to a purpose or use.'[19]

Asocial. 'Not social; indifferent to social values; without social meaning or significance.'[20]

Attention and concentration. 'The aspect of consciousness that relates to the amount of effort exerted in focusing on certain aspects of an experience.'[21]

Attitude. The 'preparatory mental posture with which one receives stimuli and reacts to them.'[22]

Awareness. 'To have perception or knowledge, conscious, informed.'[23]

Behaviour. 'The manner in which anything acts or operates. With regard to the human being the term usually refers to the action of the individual as a unit. He may be, and ordinarily is, acting in response to some given organ or impulse, but it is his general reaction that gives rise to the concept of behaviour.'[24]

Body image. 'The concept that each person has of his own body as an object in space, independently and apart from all other objects.'[25]

Body language. 'The system by which a person expresses his thoughts and feelings by means of his bodily activity.'[26]

Closed system. 'A system which does not interact with its environment or exhibit properties of life.'[27]

Cognitive functions. 'Referring to the mental process of comprehension, judgement, memory, and reasoning, as contrasted with emotional and volitional processes. Contrast with **Conative**.'[28]

Communication. The 'transmission of emotions, attitudes, ideas, and acts from one person to another. The distinction is made between the "primary" techniques of communication common to all men, such as language, gesture, the imitation of overt behaviour and social suggestion, and the "secondary" techniques which facilitate communication, such as writing, symbolic systems including stop-and-go lights, bugle-calls and other signals, and physical conditions allowing for communication such as the telephone, railroad and the airplane.'[29]

Communication/interaction skills. 'Abilities for sharing and receiving information and for coordinating one's behaviour with that of others in order to accomplish mutual activities and goals.'[30]

Communication, nonverbal. See **Nonverbal interaction**.

Communication, verbal. See **Verbalization** or **Verbal technique**.

Competence. 'The quality of being able or having the capacity to respond effectively to the demands of one or a range of situations.'[31]

Comprehension. 'Understanding, especially as opposed to mere apprehending or cognition.'[32]

Conative. 'Pertains to the basic strivings of an individual as expressed in his behaviour and actions; volitional as contrasted with cognitive.'[33]

Concentration. See **Attention**.

Conflict. 'A mental struggle that arises from the simultaneous operation of opposing impulses, drives, or external (environmental) or internal drives; termed intrapsychic when the conflict is between forces within the personality; extrapsychic when it is between the self and the environment.'[34]

Confrontation. 'Act of letting a person know where one stands in relationship to him, what one is experiencing, and how one perceives him.'[35]

Confusion. 'Disturbed orientation in respect of time, place, or person.'[36] See **Mental status**.

Conscious. 'That part of the mind or mental functioning of which the content is subject to awareness or known to the person. In neurology: awake, alert.'[37] Contrast with **Unconscious**.

Contraindication. 'A reason for not doing something; more specifically, a feature or complication of a condition that countermands the use of a therapeutic agent that might otherwise be applied.'[38]

Conversation. 'An informal talking together.'[39]

Cooperation. 'Acting jointly with another or others.'[40]

Coordination. 'Harmonious action, as of muscles.'[41]

Creativity. The 'ability to produce something new. Silvano Arieti describes creativity as the tertiary process, a balanced continuation of primary and secondary processes, whereby materials from the id are used in the service of the ego.'[42]

Debility. 'Weakness.'[43]

Decision. 'The act of making up one's mind; the act of forming an opinion or deciding upon a course of action.'[44]

Defence mechanism. 'Unconscious intrapsychic processes serving to provide relief from emotional conflict and anxiety. Conscious efforts are frequently made for the same reasons, but true defence mechanisms are unconscious. Some common defence mechanisms are: compensation, conversion, denial, displacement, dissociation, idealization, identification, incorporation, introjection, projection, rationalization, reaction formation, regression, sublimation, substitution, symbolization, undoing.'[45] See **Mental mechanism**.

Delusion. 'A firm, fixed idea not amenable to rational explanation. Maintained against logical argument despite objective contradictory evidence. Common delusions include:

delusions of grandeur: exaggerated ideas of one's importance or identity.

delusions of persecution: ideas that one has been singled out for persecution. See also **Paranoia.**

delusions of reference: incorrect assumption that certain casual or unrelated events or the behaviour of others apply to oneself.'[46]

Dependency. 'Relying on another for support.'[47]

Depression. A clinical syndrome consisting of a lowering of mood tone, loss of interest or pleasure, psychomotor retardation or agitation and difficulty in thinking or concentrating.'[48]

Dialogue. 'A conversation between two or more parties.'[49] Compare with **Monologue.**

Disappointment. 'A state of unfulfilled expectation or hope.'[50]

Discuss. 'To argue or consider carefully by presenting the various sides.'[51]

Discussion. 'The act of discussing things.'[52]

Distractibility. 'Inability to focus one's attention.'[53]

Dyssemia. 'Difficulty in using and understanding nonverbal signs and signals.'[54]

Dystonia. 'Abnormal positioning or spasm of the muscles of the head, neck, limbs or trunk developing within a few days of starting neuroleptic medication.'[55]

Ego. 'In psychoanalytic theory … the ego represents the sum of certain mental mechanisms, such as perception and memory, and specific defence mechanisms. The ego serves to mediate between the demands of primitive instinctual drives (the id), of internalized parental and social prohibitions (the superego), and of reality. The compromises between these forces achieved by the ego tend to resolve intrapsychic conflict and serve as an adaptive and executive function.'[56]

Egocentric. 'Refers to a person who is self-centred, preoccupied with his own needs, selfish and lacking interest in others.'[57]

Ego-strength. 'The effectiveness with which the ego discharges its various functions. A strong ego will not only mediate between id, superego, and reality and integrate these functions, but further it will do so with enough flexibility so that energy will remain for reactivity and other needs. This is in contrast to the rigid personality in which ego functions are maintained, but only at the cost of impoverishment of the personality.'[58]

Emotion. 'A feeling such as fear, anger, grief, joy or love which may not always be conscious.'[59] See also **Affect** and **Feeling**.

Empathy. 'An objective and insightful awareness of the feelings, emotions, and behaviour of another person, their meaning and significance; usually subjective and noncritical.'[60] Contrast with **Sympathy**.

Environment. 'The objects, persons and events with which a system interacts.'[61]

Evaluate. 'To appraise.'[62]

Exercise. 'Repetition of an act in order to learn it or increase skill.'[63]

Expectations of success or failure. 'One's anticipation of future endeavours and whether their outcomes will be successful or not.'[64]

Experiencing. 'Feeling emotions and feelings as opposed to thinking; being involved in what is happening, rather than standing back at a distance and theorizing.'[65]

Extemporaneous. 'Not planned beforehand.'[66]

External and internal locus of control. 'The individual's conviction that outcomes in life are related to personal actions (internal control) versus the action of others, fate or luck (external control).'[67]

Eye-contact. Describes the mutual glances that occur between people during social interaction. The degree of eye-contact depends on such factors as whether the participants like one another, how involved they are in their discussion, the nature of the topic under discussion and their physical position in relation to one another. The degree of eye-contact may also follow a cultural pattern that presumes touching, no touch, interpersonal spacing and the way people orient their bodies. 'Eye contact is necessary for the exchange of all visual, nonverbal information.'[68]

Feedback. 'The process of returning to the system information concerning output and its consequences.'[69] Communication to the sender of the effect his original message had on those to whom it was relayed. Feedback may alter or re-enforce the original idea; it is a function that is basic to correction and self-correction.'[70]

Feeling. '(1) Subjective description for awareness of bodily (neutral) states that cannot be reliably referred to environmental wants. (2) Tactile sensation. (3) Awareness of something, i.e. feeling of being accepted. (4) Emotion, e.g. feeling happy, sad, angry, etc.'[71]

Flight of ideas. 'Verbal skipping from one idea to another. The ideas appear to be continuous but are fragmentary and determined by chance or temporal associations. Sometimes seen in manic-depressive psychosis.'[72]

Focus. 'Focus attention on a problem.'[73]

Gesture. 'Gestures involve the use of hand and intricate finger positions in order to express an array of emotions and information.'[74]

Goal. 'Aim, purpose.'[75]

Group cohesion. 'Effect of the mutual bonds between members of a group as a result of their concentrated effort for a common interest and purpose. Until cohesiveness is achieved, the group cannot concentrate its full energy on a common task.'[76]

Group pressure. 'Demand by group members that individual members submit and conform to group standards, values and behaviour.'[77]

Habit organization. 'The degree to which one has a typical use of time which supports competent performance in a variety of environments and roles and provides a balance of activity.'[78]

Habits. 'Images guiding the routine and typical ways in which a person performs.'[79]

Habituation subsystem. 'A collection of images which trigger and guide the performance of routine patterns of behaviour.'[80]

Hallucination. 'A false sensory perception in the absence of an actual external stimulus. May be induced by emotional and other factors, such as drugs, alcohol and stress. May occur in any of the senses.'[81]

Honesty. 'In therapy, honesty is a value manifested by the ability to communicate one's immediate experience, including inconsistent, conflicting or ambivalent feelings and perceptions.'[82]

Hyperactive. 'Excessively or abnormally active.'[83]

Id. 'In Freudian theory, that part of the personality structure which harbours the unconscious instinctual desires and strivings of the individual.'[84] See **Ego** and **Superego**.

Identity-crises. 'A loss of the sense of sameness and historical continuity of one's self, an inability to accept or adopt the role the subject perceives as being expected of him by society; often expressed by isolation, withdrawal, extremism, rebelliousness, and negativity, and typically triggered by a combination of sudden increases in the strength of instinctual drives in a milieu of rapid social evolution and technological change.'[85]

Improvisation. 'In psychodrama, the acting out of problems without prior preparation;'[86] to perform or act on the spur of the moment without any preparation.

Impulse. 'A psychic striving; usually refers to an instinctual urge.'[87]

Indecision. 'A wavering between two or more possible courses of action.'[88]

Individual. 'Jung defines the psychological individual as a "unique being". The psychological individual is characterized by its peculiar, and in certain respects, unique psychology.'[89]

Individuation. 'The process of forming and specializing the individual nature; in particular, it is the development of the psychological individual as a differentiated being from the general, collective psychology.'[90]

Inhibition. 'In psychiatry, an unconscious defence against forbidden instinctual drives; it may interfere with or restrict specific activities or general patterns of behaviour.'[91]

Insight. 'Self-understanding. The extent of the individual's understanding of the origin, nature, and mechanisms of his attitudes and behaviour. More superficially, recognition by a patient that he is ill.'[92] 'Most therapists distinguish two types: (1) intellectual insight: knowledge and awareness without any change of maladaptive behaviour; (2) emotional or visceral insight: awareness, knowledge, and understanding of one's own maladaptive behaviour, leading to positive changes in personality and behaviour.'[93]

Intake. 'The importation of energy and information from the environment.'[94]

Intelligence. 'According to Thorndike, there are three distinct types of intelligence; abstract, mechanical and social. The capacity to understand and manage abstract ideas and symbols constitutes abstract intelligence; the ability to understand, invent and manage mechanisms comprises mechanical intelligence; and the capacity to act reasonably and wisely as regards human relations and social affairs constitutes social intelligence.'[95]

Intelligence quotient. 'The score obtained from one of various intelligence tests. This score is calculated for an individual in comparison with the so-called average or normal intelligence for his age. The tests measure "abstracting ability, reasoning, speed of visual information processing and many other formal cognitive processes." Aside from this cognitive factor, the I.Q. score is also influenced by motivation and achievement factors.'[96]

Inter-(*Lat.*) 'Prefix. Among other things.'[97]

Interact. 'To engage in mutual or reciprocal action.'[98]

Interaction. See **Social interaction** and **Nonverbal interaction**.

Interests. Dispositions to find occupations pleasurable.[99]

Interpersonal relations. 'Relating to or involving relations between persons.'[100]

Interpersonal skill. 'Ability of a person in relationship with others to express his feelings appropriately, to be socially responsive, to change and influence, and to work and create.'[101] See **Socialization**.

Intrapsychic. See **Conflict**.

Isolation. 'A defence mechanism, operating unconsciously, in which an unacceptable impulse, idea, or act is separated from its original memory source, thereby removing the emotional charge associated with the original memory.'[102] 'Isolation may (also) be defined as a lack of family and social contacts' and as such it 'has to be distinguished from loneliness, although the two often coexist.'[103]

Judgement. 'Mental act of comparing or evaluating choices within the framework of a given set of values for the purpose of selecting a course of action. Judgement is said to be intact if the course of action chosen is consistent with reality. Judgement is said to be impaired if the chosen course of action is not consistent with reality.'[104]

Kinesics (kinesiology). 'The study of body movement as part of the process of communication; sociological analysis of interactional activity.'[105] Kinesics includes the study of body posture, movement and facial expression.

Labile. 'Unstable, characterized by rapidly changing emotions.'[106]

Leadership. 'The role taken to direct the operations' activity or performance'[107]

Leadership role. 'Stance adopted by the therapist in conducting a group. There are three main leadership roles: authoritarian, democratic, and laissez-faire. Any group – social, therapeutic, training or task-oriented – is primarily influenced by the role practised by the leader.'[108]

Mania. 'A mood disorder characterized by excessive elation, hyper-activity, agitation, and accelerated thinking and speaking, sometimes manifested in a flight of ideas. Mania is seen most frequently as one of the two major forms of manic-depression psychosis.'[109]

Manic-depression psychosis. 'A major affective disorder characterized by severe mood swings and a tendency to remission and recurrence.'[110] See also **Depression.**

Medium. 'A condition or environment in which something may function or flourish.'[111]

Memory. 'Ability to revive past sensory impressions, experiences and learned ideas. Memory includes three basic mental processes: *registration*: the ability to perceive, recognize and establish information in the central nervous system; *retention*: the ability to retain registered information; and *recall*: the ability to retrieve stored information at will.'[112]

Mental disorder. 'Any psychiatric illness or disease included in the World Health Organization's *International Classification of Diseases.*'[113]

Mental mechanism. 'A generic term for a variety of psychic processes that are functions of the ego and largely unconscious. Includes perception, memory, thinking and defence mechanisms.'[114]

Mental status. 'The level and style of functioning of the psyche, used in its broadest sense to include intellectual functioning as well as the emotional, attitudinal, psychological and personality aspects of the subject; in clinical psychiatry, the term is commonly used to refer to the results of the examination of the patient's mental state. Such an examination ordinarily aims to achieve one or more of the following:

(1) evaluation and assessment of any psychiatric condition present, including provisional diagnosis and prognosis, determination of degree of impairment, suitability for treatment, and indications for particular types of therapeutic intervention.

(2) formulation of the personality structure of the subject, which may suggest the historical and developmental antecedents of whatever psychiatric condition exists;

(3) estimate of the ability and willingness of the subject to participate appropriately in the treatment regimen considered desirable for him. The mental status is reported in a series of narrative statements describing such things as: affect, speech, thought content, perceptions, and cognitive functions, including orientation.'[115]

Mime. 'To act or play a part, usually without words; a farce using funny actions and gestures, and the ludicrous representation of familiar types and events.'[116]

Monologue. 'A dramatic soliloquy; a long speech monopolizing conversation'.[117]

Mood. The 'feeling tone that is experienced by a person internally. Mood does not include the external expression of the internal feeling tone.'[118] See also **Affect.**

Motivation. The 'force that pushes a person to act to satisfy a need. It implies an incentive or desire that influences the will and causes the person to act.'[119]

Neologism. 'Neologisms are part of the speech disturbance which reflects the disordered thoughts of schizophrenics. They are words of the patient's own making, often condensations of other words and having a special meaning for the patient.'[120]

Neuroleptics. See **Antipsychotic agents.**

Neurosis (psychoneurosis). 'An emotional maladaptation arising from an unresolved unconscious conflict. The anxiety is either felt directly or modified by various psychological mechanisms to produce other, subjectively distressing symptoms. The neuroses are usually considered less severe than the psychoses (although not always less disabling) because they manifest neither gross personality disorganization nor gross distortion or misinterpretation of external reality. The neuroses are classified according to predominating symptoms. The common neuroses are: anxiety neurosis, depersonalization neurosis, depressive neurosis, hypochondriacal neurosis, hysterical neurosis (a) conversion type, or (b) dissociative type, neurasthenic neurosis, obsessive compulsive neurosis, phobic neurosis.'[121]

Nonverbal interaction. 'The ability to communicate nonverbal information through facial expressions, postures, gestures, interpersonal distance, tone of voice, clothing and the like.'[122]

Objectics. 'Refers to our style of dress and the other ways in which we communicate to others through our appearance. They include such things as cosmetics, jewelry, hairstyles, perfumes, deodorants and clothing.'[123]

Objective. 'Treating or dealing with facts without distortion by personal feelings or prejudices.'[124]

Observation. 'The act of gathering of information by noting facts or occurrences.'[125]

Obsessive-compulsive (psycho) neurosis. 'A type of psychoneurosis characterized by disturbing, unwanted, anxiety-provoking, intruding thoughts or ideas, and repetitive impulses to perform acts (ceremonials, counting, hand-washing, etc.) which may be considered abnormal, undesirable or distasteful to the patient.'[126]

Open system. 'A composition of interrelated structures and functions organized into a coherent whole that interacts with an environment and that is capable of maintaining and changing itself.'[127]

Opinion. 'A belief stronger than impression and less strong than positive knowledge.'[128]

Optimum. 'The amount or degree of something most favourable to an end.'[129]

Orientation. 'Awareness of one's self in relation to time, place and person.'[130]

Output. 'The action of the system directed at the environment.'[131]

Overinclusion. 'Overinclusive thinking is one aspect of thought disorder in acute schizophrenia. There is an inability to preserve conceptual boundaries, so that ideas only distantly related to a particular concept become included in that concept. The "wooliness" of schizophrenic thought is a result of this type of thought disorder.'[132]

Paralanguage. 'Refers to all the aspects of sound which accompany words or act independently of them to communicate emotion. Included are such things as tone, loudness, intensity of voice, and the sounds such as humming and whistling which are uttered between or instead of words.'[133]

Paranoid. 'An adjective applied to individuals who are overly suspicious.'[134]

Parkinsonism. See **Tremor**.

Participation. 'The action of taking part in something.'[135] See also **Activity**.

Passivity. 'One of the several modalities of adaptation. For example, it is possible for the organism to adapt itself to its environment by going either forward to meet it or backward to escape it. The first procedure would be termed the modality of activity in adaptive behaviour, while the latter would be termed the modality of passivity.'[136]

Perception. 'Mental processes by which data – intellectual, sensory and emotional – are organized meaningfully. Through perception a person makes sense out of the many stimuli that bombard him. It is one of the many ego functions.'[137]

Perceptual expansion. 'Development of one's ability to recognize and interpret the meaning of sensory stimuli through associations with past experiences with similar stimuli. Perceptual expansion through the relaxation of defences is one of the goals of both individual and group therapy.'[138]

Perceptual motor skills. 'Abilities for interpreting sensory information and for manipulating self and objects.'[139]

Performance subsystem. 'A collection of images and biological structures and processes which are organized into skills and used in the production of purposeful behaviour.'[140]

Personal causation. 'A collection of beliefs and expectations which a person holds about his or her effectiveness in the environment.'[141]

Personal space. 'Refers to the portable territory we all carry around with us. It is often depicted as a flexible bubble which is wider in the back than in the front and contracts or expands depending on the situation.'[142]

Personality. 'The characteristic way in which a person behaves; the ingrained pattern of behaviour that each person evolves, both consciously and unconsciously, as his style of life or way of being in adapting to his environment.'[143] See also **Personality disorders.**

Personality disorders. 'A group of mental disorders characterized by deeply ingrained maladaptive patterns of behaviour, generally life-long in duration and consequently often recognizable by the time of adolescence or earlier. Affecting primarily the personality of the individual they are different in quality from neurosis and psychosis.'[144]

Philosophy. 'A critical study of fundamental beliefs and the grounds for them.'[145]

Problem. 'A question raised for consideration or solution: an intricate unsettled question.'[146]

Process skills. 'Abilities directed at managing events or processes in the environment.'[147]

Projection. 'Unconscious defence mechanism in which a person attributes to another the ideas, thoughts, feelings, and impulses that are part of his inner perceptions but that are unacceptable to him. Projection protects the person from anxiety arising from an inner conflict. By externalizing whatever is unacceptable, the person deals with it as a situation apart from himself.'[148]

Projective techniques. 'Methods used to discover an individual's attitudes, motivations, defensive manoeuvres and characteristic ways of responding through analysis of their responses to unstructured, ambiguous stimuli.'[149] As a group treatment procedure they may make use of the spontaneous creative work of each patient. For example, group members make and analyse drawings, which in turn often express their underlying emotional problems.

Psychiatry. 'The medical science that deals with the origin, diagnosis, prevention and treatment of mental disorders.'[150]

Psychomotor. 'Relating to voluntary movement.'[151]

Psychomotor retardation. 'A generalized "retardation" of physical and emotional reactions.'[152]

Psychosis. 'A major mental disorder of organic or emotional origin in which the individual's ability to think, respond emotionally, remember, communicate, interpret reality, and behave appropriately is sufficiently impaired so as to interfere grossly with his capacity to meet the ordinary demands of life. Often characterized by regressive behaviour, inappropriate mood, diminished impulse control, and such abnormal mental content as delusions and hallucinations. The term is applicable to conditions having a wide range of severity and duration.'[153] See **Schizophrenia, Manic-depressive psychosis, Depression** and **Reality testing.**

Purpose. See **Goal.**

Reaction(s). 'Counter-action; response to a stimulus.'[154]

Reality. 'The totality of objective things and factual events. Reality includes everything that is perceived by a person's special senses and is validated by other people.'[155]

Reality, control with. See **Reality testing.**

Reality testing. A 'fundamental ego function that consists of objective evaluation and judgement of the world outside the self. By interacting with his animate and inanimate environment, a person tests its real nature, as well as his own relation to it. How the person evaluates reality and his attitudes towards it are determined by early experiences with significant persons in his life.'[156] 'The ability to evaluate the external world objectively and differentiate adequately between it and the internal world, between self and non-self. Falsification of reality, as with massive denial or projection, indicates a severe disturbance of ego functioning and/or the perceptual and memory processes upon which it is partly based.'[157] See also **Ego** and **Psychosis.**

Recall. 'The process of bringing memory into consciousness.' In psychiatry, 'recall is often used to refer to the recollection of facts and events in the immediate past.'[158] See **Memory.**

Recognition. 'The state of being recognized: special notice or attention.'[159]

Relatedness. 'The interrelation between two or more people who reciprocally influence each other, as patient–therapist, mother–child, etc. Normal relatedness is based on security in interpersonal relations and in large part is a result of early childhood experiences.'[160]

Relatedness, functional. 'The arrangement of objects that are organically and dynamically related to each other; for example, placing woodworking tools near the woodworking bench and nails and other objects involved in woodworking nearby; placing drawing paper near crayons and paints in the proximity of an easel.'[161]

Relaxation. 'Diminution of tension.'[162]

Repression. 'A defence mechanism, operating unconsciously, that banishes unacceptable ideas, affects or impulses from consciousness, or that keeps out of consciousness what has never been conscious. Although not subject to voluntary recall, the repressed material may emerge in disguised form. Often confused with the conscious mechanism of suppression.'[163]

Resistance. 'The individual's conscious or unconscious psychological defence against bringing repressed (unconscious) thoughts to light.'[164] See **Mental mechanism.**

Retardation. 'Slowness or backwardness of intellectual development; when used in this sense, mental retardation is the usual phrase. Slowness of response, a slowing down of thinking and/or a decrease in psychomotor activity; in this latter sense, the term psychomotor retardation is the appropriate phrase. Psychomotor retardation is characteristic of clinical depressions.'[165]

Risk. 'Exposure to possible loss or injury; danger or peril.'[166]

Role. 'Pattern of behaviour that a person takes. It has its roots in childhood and is influenced by significant people with whom the person has primary relationships. When the behaviour pattern conforms with the expectations and demands of other people, it is said to be a complementary role. If it does not conform with the demands and expectations of others, it is known as a non-complementary role.'[167]

Role balance. Integration of an optimal number of appropriate roles into one's life.'[168]

Role-playing. 'Psychodrama technique in which a person is trained to function more effectively in his reality roles, such as employer, employee, student or instructor.'[169]

Schizophrenia. 'A large group of disorders, usually of psychotic proportion, manifested by characteristic disturbances of thought, mood and behaviour. Thought disturbances are marked by alterations of concept formation that may lead to misinterpretation of reality and sometimes to delusions and hallucinations. Mood changes include ambivalence, constriction, inappropriateness, and loss of empathy with others. Behaviour may be withdrawn, regressive, and bizarre.'[170]

Sedentary. '(1) Used in sitting. (2) Related to the habit of sitting.'[171]

Self-analysis. 'Investigation of one's own psychic components.'[172]

Self-assertion. 'Self-assurance, boldness.'[173]

Self-awareness. 'Sense of knowing what one is experiencing; for example, realizing that one has responded with anger to another group member as a substitute for the anxiety left when he attacked a vital part of one's self-concept. Self-awareness is a major goal of all therapy, individual or group.'[174]

Self-conception. An individual's self-conception is his view of himself. Self-conception is the equivalent to the self, if the latter is defined as 'the individual as perceived by that individual in a socially determined form of reference.' In addition to a view of self, self-conception includes notions of one's interests and aversions, a conception of one's goals and success in achieving them, a picture of the ideological frame of reference through which one views oneself and other objects and some knowledge of self-evaluation.

Self-confidence. 'Belief in one's own ability, power or judgement.'[175]

Self-consciousness. 'Uncomfortable consciousness of oneself as an object of observation by others.'[176]

Self-esteem. 'To have a high regard or value for oneself.'[177]

Self-respect. 'To consider oneself deserving of high regard.'[178] See **Self-esteem.**

Sensory. 'Relating to or conducting sensation.'[179]

Sensory/motor functions. Skill and performance patterns of sensory and motor behaviour that are prerequisites to self-care, work and play/leisure performance. Components are neuromuscular and sensory integrative skills.

Serotonin. 'A neurotransmitter hypothesized as being involved in the production of affective disorders.'[180]

Skills. 'The abilities that a person has for the performance of various forms of purposeful behaviour.'[181]

Social isolation. See **Isolation.**

Socialization. Adaptation to social needs or uses; active participation in social gatherings.'[182]

Sociofugal. 'When the semi-fixed features of a room such as tables and chairs are arranged to discourage interaction.'[183]

Sociopetal. 'When the semi-fixed features of a room such as tables and chairs are arranged to encourage interaction.'[184]

Spontaneous. 'Acting or taking place without external force or cause, syn: impulsive, instinctive, automatic, unpremeditated.'[185]

Stimulation. See **Activation.**

Structured group. 'One in which the leaders structure the environment in an active and supportive way in order to ensure maximum participation of all members.'[186]

Subjective. 'Of or relating to, or arising within oneself or mind in contrast to what is outside.'[187]

Superego. 'In psychoanalytic theory, that part of the personality structure associated with ethics, standards and self-criticism. It is formed by the infant's identification with important and esteemed persons in his early life, particularly parents. The supposed or actual wishes of these significant persons are taken over as part of the child's own personal standards to help form the conscience.'[188] See also **Ego** and **Id.**

Support, to. 'To back, assist, uphold, advocate, champion.'[189]

Supportive psychotherapy. 'A type of psychotherapy that aims to reinforce a patient's defences and to help him suppress disturbing psychological material. Supportive psychotherapy utilizes such measures as inspiration, reassurance, suggestion, persuasion, counselling and re-education. It avoids probing the patient's emotional conflicts in depth.'[190]

Suppression. 'The conscious effort to control and conceal unacceptable impulses, thoughts, feelings, or acts.'[191]

Symbolization. 'An unconscious mental process operating by association and based on similarity and abstract representation whereby one subject or idea comes to stand for another through some part, quality or aspect which the two have in common. The symbol carries in more or less disguised form the emotional feelings vested in the initial object or idea.'[192]

Sympathy. 'Compassion for another's grief or loss. To be differentiated from empathy.'[193]

Tactile. 'Relating to the sense of touch.'[194]

Tardive dyskinesia. 'Involuntary choreiform athetoid or rhythmic move-ments (lasting at least a few weeks) of the tongue, jaw or extremities developing in association with the use of neuroleptic medication for at least a few months.'[195]

Temporal orientation. The degree to which a task is time-limiting or continuous, and seasonal or discretionary.[196]

Tension. 'An unpleasant alteration of affect characterized by a strenuous increase in mental and physical activity.'[197]

Theatre game. A simple, structured exercise, often used by actors to improve their abilities to think quickly, to be spontaneous, to improvise, to speak clearly, to trust others, to work in cooperation with others, to concentrate and to be decisive. The emphasis in a theatre game is upon clear, direct communication, whether it be verbal or nonverbal, and if it is used appropriately and in conjunc-tion with other theatre games it can offer an excellent opportunity to practise, improve or change social behaviour in an enjoyable and accepting atmosphere.

Therapeutic. 'To attend, treat, related to or dealing with healing and especially with remedies.'[198]

Thinking, abstract. 'Thinking which is characterized by the use of abstractions and generalizations.'[199]

Thinking, concrete. The antithesis of abstract thinking. Concrete thinking is often associated with impairment of the frontal lobes. It is characterized by 'an inability to detach the ego from the inner and outer sphere of experience; an inability to concentrate on two tasks simultaneously; to integrate parts into a whole or to analyse a totality; and an inability to judge, reflect about or plan for the future.'[200]

Throughput. 'The transformation of imported information and energy to another form and its incorporation into the structure of the system resulting in structural maintenance and change.'[201]

Tremor. 'Shaking or trembling. A disorder of muscular tone in which the usual, normal, unappreciable tonic contractions of a muscle become exaggerated to the point of awareness. In general, tremors can be classified into:

(1) coarse tremors, usually indicative of organic disease; included are:

(a) passive or rest tremor, a tremor that occurs while the affected area is at rest, as the pill-rolling tremor of Parkinsonism;
(b) action or intention tremor, which may be absent while the affected area is at rest and which is exaggerated by voluntary movement of the area, as the intention tremor of multiple sclerosis;

(2) fine tremors, often psychogenic, although they may also be on toxic basis (alcoholism, drug-poisoning hyperthyroidism, etc.);

(3) fasciculation, involuntary twitchings of a portion of a muscle; seen in fatigue, also in brain stem or anterior horn cell damage.'[202]

Trust, basic. 'The basis of reliance, faith or hope.'[203]

Unconscious. 'That part of the mind or mental functioning of which the content is only rarely subject to awareness. It is the repository for data that have never been conscious (primary repression) or that may have become conscious briefly and later repressed (secondary repression).'[204]

Values. 'Images of what is good, right and/or important.'[205]

Verbalization. 'In psychiatry, the state of being verbose or diffuse, commonly encountered in extreme degree in patients with the manic form of manic-depressive psychosis. In a more general sense, verbalization refers to the expression in words of thoughts, wishes, fantasies, or other psychic material which had previously been on a nonverbal level because of suppression. "Verbalize" is often used in a pseudoerudite way when "talk about" is meant.'[206]

Verbal technique. 'Any method of group or individual therapy in which words are used.'[207]

Videotape. 'To make a recording of visual images and sound on a magnetic tape.'[208]

Volition sub-system. 'An interrelated set of energizing and symbolic components which together determine conscious choices for occupational behaviour.'[209]

Warm-up exercise. 'A technique, exercise or game of short duration used to promote an atmosphere in which individuals can begin to look at specific problems in general detail.'[210]

Withdrawal. 'The act of retracting, retiring, retreating or going away from. Withdrawal is used in psychiatry to refer to ... the turning away from objective, external reality ... the patient's retreat from society and interpersonal relationships into a world of his own.'[211] Often seen in schizophrenia and depression.

Word salad. 'A mixture of words and/or phrases which have no logical meaning. Commonly associated with schizophrenia.'[212]

REFERENCES

1. *The Merriam-Webster Dictionary* (1997), p. 23, Springfield, Massachusetts.
2. Frazier, S. H., Campbell, R. J., Marshall, M. H., Werner, A. (1975) *A Psychiatric Glossary*, p. 10. New York: Basic Books.
3. Hinsie, L. E., Campbell, R. J. (1970) *Psychiatric Dictionary*, 4th edn., p. 12. New York: Oxford University Press.
4. Freedman, A. M., Kaplan, A. I., Sadock, B. J. (Eds.) (1972) *Modern Synopsis of Psychiatry*, p. 749. Baltimore: Williams & Wilkins.
5. Hinsie, L. E., Campbell, R. J. (1970) *Psychiatric Dictionary*, 4th edn., p. 13. New York: Oxford University Press.
6. *Ibid*, p. 13.
7. *Ibid*, p. 14.
8. Frazier, S. H., Campbell, R. J., Marshall, M. H., Werner, A. (1975) *A Psychiatric Glossary*, p. 11. New York: Basic Books.

9. Freedman, A. M., Kaplan, A. I., Sadock, B. J. (1976) *Modern Synopsis of Comprehensive Textbook of Psychiatry/II*, 2nd edn, p. 1280. Baltimore: Williams & Wilkins.

10. Frazier, S. H., Campbell, R. J., Marshall, M. H., Werner, A. (1975) *A Psychiatric Glossary*, p. 11. New York: Basic Books.

11. *Ibid*, p. 13.

12. *The Merriam-Webster Dictionary* (1997), p. 45, Springfield, Massachusetts.

13. Ralph, I. (1996) *Psychotropic Agents. Handbook for Mental Health Workers*, p. 2. Delta, B. C.: IGR Publications.

14. *Ibid*, p. 2.

15. Frazier, S. H., Campbell, R. J., Marshall, M. H., Werner, A. (1975) *A Psychiatric Glossary*, p. 16. New York: Basic Books.

16. Freedman, A. M., Kaplan, A. I., Sadock, B. J. (Eds.) (1972) *Modern Synopsis of Psychiatry*, p. 753. Baltimore: Williams & Wilkins.

17. Wolman, Benjamin I. (1973) *Dictionary of Behavioural Science*, p. 29. New York: Litton Educational Publishing.

18. Hinsie, L. E., Campbell, R. J. (1970) *Psychiatric Dictionary*, 4th edn., pp. 59–60. New York: Oxford University Press.

19. *The Merriam-Webster Dictionary* (1997), p. 52, Springfield, Massachusetts.

20. Hinsie, L. E., Campbell, R. J. (1970) *Psychiatric Dictionary*, 4th edn., p. 66. New York: Oxford University Press.

21. Freedman, A. M., Kaplan, A. I., Sadock, B. J. (Eds.) (1972) *Modern Synopsis of Psychiatry*, p. 754. Baltimore: Williams & Wilkins.

22. *Ibid*, p. 754.

23. *The Merriam-Webster Dictionary* (1997), p. 67, Springfield, Massachusetts.

24. Hinsie, L. E., Campbell, R. J. (1970) *Psychiatric Dictionary*, 4th edn., p. 90. New York: Oxford University Press.

25. Campbell, R. J. (1989) *Psychiatric Dictionary*, p. 355, Oxford, Oxford University Press.

26. Freedman, A. M., Kaplan, A. I., Sadock, B. J. (1976) *Modern Synopsis of Comprehensive Textbook of Psychiatry/II*, 2nd edn, p. 1286. Baltimore: Williams & Wilkins.

27. Kielhofner, G. (Ed.) (1985) *A Model of Human Occupation, Theory and Application*, p. 502. Baltimore: Williams & Wilkins.

28. Frazier, S. H., Campbell, R. J., Marshall, M. H., Werner, A. (1975) *A Psychiatric Glossary*, p. 33. New York: Basic Books.

29. Hinsie, L. E., Campbell, R. J. (1960) *Psychiatric Dictionary*, 3rd edn., p. 135. New York: Oxford University Press.

30. Kielhofner, G. (Ed.) (1985) *A Model of Human Occupation, Theory and Application*, p. 502. Baltimore: Williams & Wilkins.

31. *Ibid*, p. 502.

32. Hinsie, L. E., Campbell, R. J. (1970) *Psychiatric Dictionary*, 4th edn., p. 147. New York: Oxford University Press.

33. Frazier, S. H., Campbell, R. J., Marshall, M. H., Werner, A. (1975) *A Psychiatric Glossary*, p. 35. New York: Basic Books.

34. Ibid, p. 36.

35. Freedman, A. M., Kaplan, A. I., Sadock, B. J. (Eds.) (1972) *Modern Synopsis of Psychiatry*, p. 756. Baltimore: Williams & Wilkins.

36. Frazier, S. H., Campbell, R. J., Marshall, M. H., Werner, A. (1975) *A Psychiatric Glossary*, p. 36. New York: Basic Books.

37. Frazier, S. H., Campbell, R. J., Marshall, M. H., Werner, A. (1975) *A Psychiatric Glossary*, p. 36. New York: Basic Books.

38. Hinsie, L. E., Campbell, R. J. (1970) *Psychiatric Dictionary*, 4th edn., p. 161. New York: Oxford University Press.

39. *The Merriam-Webster Dictionary* (1997), p. 176, Springfield, Massachusetts.

40. *Ibid*, p. 177.

41. *The Faber Medical Dictionary* (1997) Sir Cecil Wakeley (Ed.) revised by Bate, J. G., p. 106, London, Faber and Faber.

42. Freedman, A. M., Kaplan, A. I., Sadock, B. J. (Eds.) (1972) *Modern Synopsis of Psychiatry*, p. 761. Baltimore: Williams & Wilkins.

43. The Faber Medical Dictionary (1975) Sir Cecil Wakeley (Ed.) revised by Bate, J. G., p. 118. London, Faber and Faber.

44. *The World Book Dictionary* (1990), p. 538. Chicago: World Book Inc.

45. Frazier, S. H., Campbell, R. J., Marshall, M. H., Werner, A. (1975) *A Psychiatric*

Glossary, p. 40. New York: Basic Books.

46. *Ibid*, p. 41.
47. *The Merriam-Webster Dictionary* (1997), p. 209, Springfield, Massachusetts.
48. Campbell, R. J. (1989) *Psychiatric Dictionary*,p.191, Oxford; Oxford University Press.
49. *The Merriam-Webster Dictionary* (1997), p. 216, Springfield, Massachusetts.
50. *Ibid*, p. 220.
51. *Ibid*, p. 222.
52. *The World Book Dictionary* (1990), p. 600. Chicago: World Book Inc.
53. Freedman, A. M., Kaplan, A. I., Sadock, B. J. (Eds.) (1972) *Modern Synopsis of Psychiatry*, p. 763. Baltimore: Williams & Wilkins.
54. Norwicki, S., Duke, M. (1992), *Helping the Child who Doesn't Fit In*, p. 19. Atlanta: Peachtree Publishers.
55. *Diagnostic and Statistical Manual of Mental Disorders.* 4th edn. (1994), p. 679. American Psychiatric Association.
56. Freedman, A. M., Kaplan, A. I., Sadock, B. J. (Eds.) (1972) *Modern Synopsis of Psychiatry*, p. 48. Baltimore: Williams & Wilkins.
57. *Ibid*, p. 765.
58. Hinsie, L. E., Campbell, R. J. (1970) *Psychiatric Dictionary*, 4th edn., p. 256. New York: Oxford University Press.
59. Frazier, S. H., Campbell, R. J., Marshall, M. H., Werner, A. (1975) *A Psychiatric Glossary*, p. 50. New York: Basic Books.
60. *Ibid*, p. 51.
61. Kielhofner, G. (Ed.) (1985) *A Model of Human Occupation, Theory and Application*, p. 503. Baltimore: Williams & Wilkins.
62. *The Merriam-Webster Dictionary* (1997), p. 262, Springfield, Massachusetts.
63. Wolman, Benjamin I. (1973) *Dictionary of Behavioural Science*, p. 131. New York: Litton Educational Publishing.
64. Kielhofner, G. (Ed.) (1985) *A Model of Human Occupation, Theory and Application*, p. 17. Baltimore: Williams & Wilkins.
65. Freedman, A. M., Kaplan, A. I., Sadock, B. J. (1976) *Modern Synopsis of Comprehensive Textbook of Psychiatry/II*, 2nd edn, p. 1300. Baltimore: Williams & Wilkins.
66. *The Merriam-Webster Dictionary* (1997), p. 268, Springfield, Massachusetts.
67. Kielhofner, G. (Ed.) (1985) *A Model of Human Occupation, Theory and Application*, p. 16. Baltimore: Williams & Wilkins.
68. Norwicki, S., Duke, M. (1992) *Helping the Child who Doesn't Fit In*, p. 85, Atlanta: Peachtree Publishers.
69. Kielhofner, G. (Ed.) (1985) *A Model of Human Occupation, Theory and Application*, p. 16. Baltimore: Williams & Wilkins.
70. Hinsie, L. E., Campbell, R. J. (1970) *Psychiatric Dictionary*, 4th edn., p. 298. New York: Oxford University Press.
71. Wolman, Benjamin I. (1973) *Dictionary of Behavioural Science*, p. 143. New York: Litton Educational Publishing.
72. Frazier, S. H., Campbell, R. J., Marshall, M. H., Werner, A. (1975) *A Psychiatric Glossary*, p. 56. New York: Basic Books.
73. *The Merriam-Webster Dictionary* (1997), p. 295, Springfield, Massachusetts.
74. Norwicki, S., Duke, M. (1992) *Helping the Child who Doesn't Fit In*, p. 66. Atlanta: Peachtree Publications.
75. *The Merriam-Webster Dictionary* (1997), p. 324, Springfield, Massachusetts.
76. Freedman, A. M., Kaplan, A. I., Sadock, B. J. (Eds.) (1972) *Modern Synopsis of Psychiatry*, p. 770. Baltimore: Williams & Wilkins.
77. Ibid, p. 770.
78. Kielhofner, G. (Ed.) (1985) *A Model of Human Occupation, Theory and Application*, p. 504. Baltimore: Williams & Wilkins.
79. *Ibid*, p. 504.
80. *Ibid*, p. 504.
81. Frazier, S. H., Campbell, R. J., Marshall, M. H., Werner, A. (1975) *A Psychiatric Glossary*, p. 61. New York: Basic Books.
82. Freedman, A. M., Kaplan, A. I., Sadock, B. J. (Eds.) (1972) *Modern Synopsis of Psychiatry*, p. 771. Baltimore: Williams & Wilkins.
83. The Faber Medical Dictionary (1975) Sir Cecil Wakeley (Ed.) revised by Bate, J. G. p. 213, London, Faber and Faber.
84. Frazier, S. H., Campbell, R. J., Marshall, M. H., Werner, A. (1975) *A Psychiatric*

Glossary, p. 64. New York: Basic Books.

85. *Ibid*, p. 65.
86. Freedman, A. M., Kaplan, A. I., Sadock, B. J. (1976) *Modern Synopsis of Comprehensive Textbook of Psychiatry/II*, 2nd edn., p. 1308. Baltimore: Williams & Wilkins.
87. Frazier, S. H., Campbell, R. J., Marshall, M. H., Werner, A. (1975) *A Psychiatric Glossary*, p. 66. New York: Basic Books.
88. *The Merriam-Webster Dictionary* (1997), p. 380, Springfield, Massachusetts.
89. Hinsie, L. E., Campbell, R. J. (1970) *Psychiatric Dictionary*, 4th edn., p. 390. New York: Oxford University Press.
90. *Ibid*, p. 390.
91. Sternberg, R. J. (1982) *Handbook of Human Intelligence*, pp. 600–601. Cambridge: Cambridge University Press.
92. Frazier, S. H., Campbell, R. J., Marshall, M. H., Werner, A. (1975) *A Psychiatric Glossary*, p. 89. New York: Basic Books.
93. Freedman, A. M., Kaplan, A. I., Sadock, B. J. (1976) *Modern Synopsis of Comprehensive Textbook of Psychiatry/II*, 2nd edn., p. 1309. Baltimore: Williams & Wilkins.
94. Kielhofner, G. (Ed.) (1985) *A Model of Human Occupation, Theory and Application*, p. 504. Baltimore: Williams & Wilkins.
95. Hinsie, L. E., Campbell, R. J. (1970) *Psychiatric Dictionary*, 4th edn., p. 406. New York: Oxford University Press.
96. *Ibid*, p. 640.
97. *The Merriam-Webster Dictionary* (1997), p. 392, Springfield, Massachusetts.
98. *Ibid,* p. 392.
99. Kielhofner, G. (Ed.) (1985) *A Model of Human Occupation, Theory and Application*, p. 504. Baltimore: Williams & Wilkins.
100. *The Merriam-Webster Dictionary* (1997), p. 392, Springfield, Massachusetts.
101. Freedman, A. M., Kaplan, A. I., Sadock, B. J. (1976) *Modern Synopsis of Comprehensive Textbook of Psychiatry/II*, 2nd edn., p. 1310. Baltimore: Williams & Wilkins.
102. Frazier, S. H., Campbell, R. J., Marshall, M. H., Werner, A. (1975) *A Psychiatric Glossary*, p. 90. New York: Basic Books.
103. Leigh, D., Pare, C. M. B., Marks, J. (Eds.) (1977) *A Concise Encyclopaedia of Psychiatry*, p. 207. Baltimore: University Park Press.
104. Freedman, A. M., Kaplan, A. I., Sadock, B. J. (1976) *Modern Synopsis of Comprehensive Textbook of Psychiatry/II*, 2nd edn., p. 1311. Baltimore: Williams & Wilkins.
105. Frazier, S. H., Campbell, R. J., Marshall, M. H., Werner, A. (1975) *A Psychiatric Glossary*, p. 92. New York: Basic Books.
106. Freedman, A. M., Kaplan, A. I., Sadock, B. J. (1976) *Modern Synopsis of Comprehensive Textbook of Psychiatry/II*, 2nd edn., p. 1312. Baltimore: Williams & Wilkins.
107. *The Merriam-Webster Dictionary* (1997), p. 423, Springfield, Massachusetts.
108. Freedman, A. M., Kaplan, A. I., Sadock, B. J. (Eds.) (1972) *Modern Synopsis of Psychiatry*, p. 777. Baltimore: Williams & Wilkins.
109. Frazier, S. H., Campbell, R. J., Marshall, M. H., Werner, A. (1975) *A Psychiatric Glossary*, p. 97. New York: Basic Books.
110. *Ibid*, p. 90.
111. *The Merriam-Webster Dictionary* (1997), p. 480, Springfield, Massachusetts.
112. Freedman, A. M., Kaplan, A. I., Sadock, B. J. (Eds.) (1972) *Modern Synopsis of Psychiatry*, p. 779. Baltimore: Williams & Wilkins.
113. Frazier, S. H., Campbell, R. J., Marshall, M. H., Werner, A. (1975) *A Psychiatric Glossary*, p. 99. New York: Basic Books.
114. *Ibid*, p. 99.
115. *Ibid*, p. 100.
116. *The World Book Dictionary* (1990), p. 1320. Chicago: World Book Inc.
117. *The Merriam-Webster Dictionary* (1997,) p. 480, Springfield, Massachusetts.
118. Freedman, A. M., Kaplan, A. I., Sadock, B. J. (1976) *Modern Synopsis of Comprehensive Textbook of Psychiatry/II*, 2nd edn., p. 1316. Baltimore: Williams & Wilkins.
119. *Ibid*, p. 1317.
120. Leigh, D., Pare, C. M. B., Marks, J. (Eds.) (1977) *A Concise Encyclopaedia of Psychiatry*, p. 254. Baltimore: University Park Press.

121. Frazier, S. H., Campbell, R. J., Marshall, M. H., Werner, A. (1975) *A Psychiatric Glossary*, p. 106. New York: Basic Books.
122. Norwicki, S., Duke, M. (1992) *Helping the Child who Doesn't Fit In*, p. 5, Atlanta: Peachtree Publications.
123. Norwicki, S., Duke, M. (1992), *Helping the Child who Doesn't Fit In*, p. 113. Atlanta: Peachtree Publishers.
124. *The Merriam-Webster Dictionary* (1997), p. 510, Springfield, Massachusetts.
125. *The Merriam-Webster Dictionary* (1997), p. 511, Springfield, Massachusetts.
126. Hinsie, L. E., Campbell, R. J. (1970) *Psychiatric Dictionary*, 4th edn., p. 519. New York: Oxford University Press.
127. Kielhofner, G. (Ed.) (1985) *A Model of Human Occupation, Theory and Application*, p. 506. Baltimore: Williams & Wilkins.
128. *The Merriam-Webster Dictionary* (1997), p. 519, Springfield, Massachusetts.
129. *Ibid*, p. 519.
130. Frazier, S. H., Campbell, R. J., Marshall, M. H., Werner, A. (1975) *A Psychiatric Glossary*, p. 111. New York: Basic Books.
131. Kielhofner, G. (Ed.) (1985) *A Model of Human Occupation, Theory and Application*, p. 506. Baltimore: Williams & Wilkins.
132. Leigh, D., Pare, C. M. B., Marks, J. (Eds.) (1977) *A Concise Encyclopaedia of Psychiatry*, p. 268. Baltimore: University Park Press.
133. Norwicki, S., Duke, M. (1992), *Helping the Child who Doesn't Fit In*, p. 97. Atlanta: Peachtree Publishers.
134. Frazier, S. H., Campbell, R. J., Marshall, M. H., Werner, A. (1975) *A Psychiatric Glossary*, p. 112. New York: Basic Books.
135. *The Merriam-Webster Dictionary* (1997), p. 537, Springfield, Massachusetts.
136. Hinsie, L. E., Campbell, R. J. (1970) *Psychiatric Dictionary*, 4th edn., p. 548. New York: Oxford University Press.
137. Freedman, A. M., Kaplan, A. I., Sadock, B. J. (1976) *Modern Synopsis of Comprehensive Textbook of Psychiatry/II*, 2nd edn., p. 1320. Baltimore: Williams & Wilkins.
138. Freedman, A. M., Kaplan, A. I., Sadock, B. J. (1976) *Modern Synopsis of Comprehensive Textbook of Psychiatry/II*, 2nd edn., p. 1320. Baltimore: Williams & Wilkins.
139. Kielhofner, G. (Ed.) (1985) *A Model of Human Occupation, Theory and Application*, p. 507. Baltimore: Williams & Wilkins.
140. *Ibid*, p. 507
141. *Ibid*, p. 507.
142. Norwicki, S., Duke, M. (1992), *Helping the Child who Doesn't Fit In*, p. 44. Atlanta: Peachtree Publishers.
143. Frazier, S. H., Campbell, R. J., Marshall, M. H., Werner, A. (1975) *A Psychiatric Glossary*, p. 115. New York: Basic Books.
144. *Ibid*, p. 116.
145. *The Merriam-Webster Dictionary* (1997), p. 552, Springfield, Massachusetts.
146. *Ibid*, p. 584.
147. Kielhofner, G. (Ed.) (1985) *A Model of Human Occupation, Theory and Application*, p. 508. Baltimore: Williams & Wilkins.
148. Freedman, A. M., Kaplan, A. I., Sadock, B. J. (1976) *Modern Synopsis of Comprehensive Textbook of Psychiatry/II*, 2nd edn., p. 1322. Baltimore: Williams & Wilkins.
149. Wolman, Benjamin I. (1973) *Dictionary of Behavioural Science*, p. 291. New York: Litton Educational Publishing.
150. Frazier, S. H., Campbell, R. J., Marshall, M. H., Werner, A. (1975) *A Psychiatric Glossary*, p. 124. New York: Basic Books.
151. Faber, p. 368.
152. Frazier, S. H., Campbell, R. J., Marshall, M. H., Werner, A. (1975) *A Psychiatric Glossary*, p. 126. New York: Basic Books.
153. *Ibid*, p. 127.
154. Hinsie, L. E., Campbell, R. J. (1970) *Psychiatric Dictionary*, 4th edn., p. 645. New York: Oxford University Press.
155. Freedman, A. M., Kaplan, A. I., Sadock, B. J. (1976) *Modern Synopsis of Comprehensive Textbook of Psychiatry/II*, 2nd edn., p. 1325. Baltimore: Williams & Wilkins.
156. Ibid, p. 1325.
157. Frazier, S. H., Campbell, R. J., Marshall, M. H., Werner, A. (1975) *A Psychiatric*

Glossary, p. 131. New York: Basic Books.
158. *Ibid*, p. 241.
159. *The Merriam-Webster Dictionary* (1997), p. 614, Springfield, Massachusetts.
160. Hinsie, L. E., Campbell, R. J. (1970) *Psychiatric Dictionary*, 4th edn., p. 658. New York: Oxford University Press.
161. *Ibid*, p. 658.
162. *The Faber Medical Dictionary* (1975) Sir Cecil Wakeley (Ed.) revised by Bate, J. G., p. 379, London, Faber and Faber.
163. Frazier, S. H., Campbell, R. J., Marshall, M. H., Werner, A. (1975) *A Psychiatric Glossary*, p. 133. New York: Basic Books.
164. *Ibid*, p. 133.
165. Hinsie, L. E., Campbell, R. J. (1970) *Psychiatric Dictionary*, 4th edn., p. 665. New York: Oxford University Press.
166. *The Merriam-Webster Dictionary* (1997), p. 638, Springfield, Massachusetts.
167. Freedman, A. M., Kaplan, A. I., Sadock, B. J. (1976) *Modern Synopsis of Comprehensive Textbook of Psychiatry/II*, 2nd edn., p. 1327. Baltimore: Williams & Wilkins.
168. Kielhofner, G. (Ed.) (1985) *A Model of Human Occupation, Theory and Application*, p. 508. Baltimore: Williams & Wilkins.
169. Freedman, A. M., Kaplan, A. I., Sadock, B. J. (1976) *Modern Synopsis of Comprehensive Textbook of Psychiatry/II*, 2nd edn., p. 1327. Baltimore: Williams & Wilkins.
170. Frazier, S. H., Campbell, R. J., Marshall, M. H., Werner, A. (1975) *A Psychiatric Glossary*, p. 134. New York: Basic Books.
171. *The Faber Medical Dictionary* (1975) Sir Cecil Wakeley (Ed.) revised by Bate, J. G., p. 396, London, Faber & Faber.
172. Freedman, A. M., Kaplan, A. I., Sadock, B. J. (1976) *Modern Synopsis of Comprehensive Textbook of Psychiatry/II*, 2nd edn., p. 1328. Baltimore: Williams & Wilkins.
173. *The Merriam-Webster Dictionary* (1997, p. 663, Springfield, Massachusetts.
174. Freedman, A. M., Kaplan, A. I., Sadock, B. J. (1976) *Modern Synopsis of Comprehensive Textbook of Psychiatry/II*, 2nd edn., p. 1328. Baltimore: Williams & Wilkins.
175. *The World Book Dictionary* (1990), p. 1887. Chicago: World Book Inc.
176. *The Merriam-Webster Dictionary* (1997), p. 663, Springfield, Massachusetts.
177. *Ibid*, p. 663.
178. *Ibid*, p. 663.
179. *The Faber Medical Dictionary* (1975) Sir Cecil Wakeley (Ed.) revised by Bate, J. G., p. 397, London, Faber & Faber.
180. Ralph, I. (1996) *Psychotropic Agents. Handbook for Mental Health Workers*, p. 73. Delta, B. C.: IGR Publications.
181. Kielhofner, G. (Ed.) (1985) *A Model of Human Occupation, Theory and Application*, p. 508. Baltimore: Williams & Wilkins.
182. *The Merriam-Webster Dictionary* (1997), p. 691, Springfield, Massachusetts.
183. Bainhart, S. A. (1976) *Introduction to Interpersonal Communication*, p. 95. New York: Thomas Y. Crowell.
184. *Ibid*, p. 95.
185. *The Merriam-Webster Dictionary* (1997), p. 702, Springfield, Massachusetts.
186. Kaplan, K. L. (1988) *Directive Group Therapy*. Thorofare, New Jersey: Slack.
187. *The Merriam-Webster Dictionary* (1997),p. 720,Springfield, Massachusetts.
188. Frazier, S. H., Campbell, R. J., Marshall, M. H., Werner, A. (1975) *A Psychiatric Glossary*, p. 143. New York: Basic Books.
189. *The Merriam-Webster Dictionary* (1997), p. 727,. Springfield, Massachusetts.
190. Frazier, S. H., Campbell, R. J., Marshall, M. H., Werner, A. (1975) *A Psychiatric Glossary*, p. 144. New York: Basic Books.
191. *Ibid*, p. 144.
192. *Ibid*, p. 144.
193. *Ibid*, p. 144.
194. *The Faber Medical Dictionary* (1975) Sir Cecil Wakeley (Ed.) revised by Bate, J. G., p. 430, London, Faber & Faber.
195. *Diagnostic and Statistical Manual of Mental Disorders*. 4th edn. (1994), p. 679. American Psychiatric Association.
196. Kielhofner, G. (Ed.) (1985) *A Model of Human Occupation, Theory and Application*, p. 509. Baltimore: Williams & Wilkins.

197. Freedman, A. M., Kaplan, A. I., Sadock, B. J. (1976) *Modern Synopsis of Comprehensive Textbook of Psychiatry/II*, 2nd edn., p. 1333. Baltimore: Williams & Wilkins.
198. *The Merriam-Webster Dictionary* (1997), p. 749, Springfield, Massachusetts.
199. Wolman, Benjamin I. (1973) *Dictionary of Behavioural Science*, p. 386. New York: Litton Educational Publishing.
200. *Ibid*, p. 386.
201. Kielhofner G. (Ed.) (1985) *A Model of Human Occupation, Theory and Application*, p. 509, Baltimore: Williams and Wilkins.
202. Hinsie, L. E., Campbell, R. J. (1970) *Psychiatric Dictionary*, 4th edn., p. 785. New York: Oxford University Press.
203. *The Merriam-Webster Dictionary* (1997), p. 777, Springfield, Massachusetts.
204. Frazier, S. H., Campbell, R. J., Marshall, M. H., Werner, A. (1975) *A Psychiatric Glossary*, p. 149. New York: Basic Books.
205. Kielhofner, G. (Ed.) (1985) *A Model of Human Occupation, Theory and Application*, p. 509. Baltimore: Williams & Wilkins.
206. Hinsie, L. E., Campbell, R. J. (1970) *Psychiatric Dictionary*, 4th edn., p. 803. New York: Oxford University Press.
207 Freedman, A. M., Kaplan, A. I., Sadock, B. J. (Eds.) (1972) *Modern Synopsis of Psychiatry*, p. 799. Baltimore: Williams & Wilkins.
208. *The Merriam-Webster Dictionary* (1997), p. 815, Springfield, Massachusetts.
209. Kielhofner, G. (Ed.) (1985) *A Model of Human Occupation, Theory and Application*, p. 509. Baltimore: Williams & Wilkins.
210. Kaplan, K.L. (1988) *Directive Group Therapy*, p.42. New Jersey: Slack Inc.
211. Hinsie, L. E., Campbell, R. J. (1970) *Psychiatric Dictionary*, 4th edn., p. 812. New York: Oxford University Press.
212. Leigh, D., Pare, C. M. B., Marks, J. (Eds.) (1977) *A Concise Encyclopaedia of Psychiatry*, p. 368. Baltimore: University Park Press.

Bibliography

This Bibliography offers some suggestions for supplementary reading; the books listed are taken from a wide variety of current publications. It invites you both to broaden your theoretical base and personal skills and to sample a greater selection of nonverbal group techniques and their potential application.

Angel, S. L. (1981) *The Emotion Identification Group.* American Journal of Occupational Therapy 35: 256.

Barris, R. (1982) *Environmental Interactions: an extension of the model of occupation.* American Journal of Occupational Therapy 36: 637

Brady, J. P. (1984) *Social Skills Training for Psychiatric Patients I: concepts, methods and clinical results.* Occupational Therapy in Mental Health 4: 51.

Brady, J. P. (1985) *Social Skills Training for Psychiatric Patients II: clinical outcome studies.* Occupational Therapy in Mental Health 5: 59.

Bruce, M., Borg, B (1987) *Frames of Reference in Psychosocial Occupational Therapy.* Thorofare, New Jersey: Charles B. Slack.

Buck, R. E., Provancher, M. A. (1972) *Magazine Picture Collages as an Evaluation Technique.* American Journal of Occupational Therapy 26: 36.

Capon, S. (1975) *Perceptual Motor Development: tire, parachute activities.* Belmont, CA: Fearon.

Creek, J. (1997) *Occupational Therapy and Mental Health.* Edinburgh: Churchill Livingstone.

Curren, D., Partridge, M., Storey, P. (1976) *Psychological Medicine: an introduction to psychiatry.* Edinburgh: Churchill Livingstone.

Cynkin, S. (1979) *Occupational Therapy: toward health through activities.* Boston: Little, Brown.

DeCarlo, J. J., Mann, W. C. (1985) *The Effectiveness of Verbal versus Activity Groups in Improving Self-perception of Interpersonal Communication Skills.* American Journal of Occupational Therapy 39: 20.

Denton, P. L. (1982) *Teaching Interpersonal Skills with Videotape.* Occupational Therapy in Mental Health 2: 17.

Denton, P. L. (1986) *Psychiatric Occupational Therapy: a workbook of practical skills.* Boston: Little, Brown.

Fluegelman, A. (1976) *The New Games Book.* San Francisco: Headlands Press.

Freedman, A. M., Kaplan, A. I., Sadock, B. J. (Eds.) (1975) *Comprehensive Textbook of Psychiatry*. Baltimore: Williams & Wilkins.

Freedman, A. M., Kaplan, H. I., Sadock, B. J. (1976) *Modern Synopsis of Comprehensive Textbook of Psychiatry/II 2nd edn.* Baltimore: Williams & Wilkins.

Harrison, R. R. (1974) *Beyond Words: an introduction to nonverbal communication*. New Jersey: Prentice Hall.

Hertzman, M. (1984) *Inpatient Psychiatry: toward rapid restoration of function*. New York: Human Services Press.

Kaplan, K. L. (1984) *Short-term Assessment: the need and a response*. Occupational Therapy in Mental Health 4(3): 29–45.

Kaplan, K. L. (1988) *Directive Group Therapy: innovative mental health treatment*. New Jersey: Slack.

Kielhofner, G. (Ed.) (1985) *A Model of Human Occupation: theory and application*. Baltimore: Williams & Wilkins.

Leigh, D., Pare, C. M. B., Marks, J. (Eds.) (1977) *A Concise Encyclopaedia of Psychiatry*. Baltimore: University Park Press.

Lerner, C. (1982) *The Magazine Picture Collage*. In: B. J. Hemphill (Ed.) *The Evaluative Process in Psychiatric Occupational Therapy*. Thorofare, New Jersey: Slack.

Moriaty, J. (1976) *Combining activities and group psychotherapy in the treatment of chronic schizophrenia*. Hospital and Community Psychiatry 27: 574–576.

Mosher, L., Keith, S. (1979) *Research on the Psychosocial Treatment of Schizophrenia*: a summary report. American Journal of Psychiatry 136: 623–631.

Norwicki, S., Duke, M. (1992) *Helping the Child who Doesn't Fit In*. Atlanta: Peachtree Publishers.

Stalker, A. (1991) *Bridges to Competence, Activities for Theme-based Social Skills Groups*. Available from the Occupational Therapy Department, British Columbia's Children's Hospital, 4480 Oak St., Vancouver, B. C., V6H 3V4, Canada.

Smith, P. B. (1980) *Group Processes and Personal Change*. London: Harper & Row.

Smith, P. B. (Ed.) (1980) *Small Groups and Personal Change*. London: Methuen.

Vandenberg, B., Kielhofner, G. (1982) *Play in Evolution, Culture and Individual Adaptation*: implications for therapy. American Journal of Occupational Therapy 36(1): 20–28.

Yalom, I. (1983) *The Lower Level Psychotherapy Group: a working model*. Inpatient Group Psychotherapy. New York: Basic Books, pp. 275–312.

Index

Entries in *italic* type indicate titles of exercises.
Page numbers in **bold** type indicate glossary entries.